Early Nutrition and
Later Achievement

Sponsored by

Centre International de l'Enfance
International Children's Centre
Centro Internacional de la Infancia

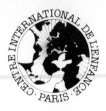

Château de Longchamp
Bois de Boulogne
75016 Paris
France

Early Nutrition and Later Achievement

Edited by

John Dobbing
Department of Child Health,
The Medical School,
University of Manchester,
England

1987

Academic Press
A Subsidiary of Harcourt Brace Jovanovich, Publishers

London   Orlando   San Diego   New York
Austin   Boston   Sydney   Tokyo   Toronto

ACADEMIC PRESS INC. (LONDON) LTD
24/28 Oval Road, London NW1 7DX

United States Edition published by
ACADEMIC PRESS INC.
Orlando, Florida 32887

British Library Cataloguing in Publication Data

Early nutrition and later achievement.
1. Health   2. Children — Nutrition
I. Dobbing, John
613′.0434   RA776.5

ISBN 0-12-218855-1

Phototypeset by
Dobbie Typesetting Limited, Plymouth, Devon

Printed in Great Britain by
St Edmundsbury Press, Bury St Edmunds, Suffolk

Contributors

D. E. Barrett, *Department of Elementary and Secondary Education, College of Education, Clemson University, Clemson, South Carolina 29634–0709, USA*

K. S. Bedi, *Department of Anatomy, University of Aberdeen, Aberdeen AB9 1AS, UK*

Linda S. Crnic, *Department of Pediatrics, University of Colorado Health Sciences Center, 4200 East 9th Avenue, Denver, Colorado 80262, USA*

J. Dobbing, *Department of Child Health, The Medical School, Oxford Road, Manchester M13 9PT, UK*

Janina R. Galler*, *Center for Behavioural Development and Mental Retardation, 85 East Newton Street, Boston, Massachusetts 02118, USA*

Sally Grantham-McGregor, *Tropical Metabolism Research Unit, University of the West Indies, Mona, Kingston 7, Jamaica, West Indies.*

I. Hurwitz*, *Department of Counseling Psychology, Boston College, Chestnut Hill, Massachusetts 02167, USA*

D. A. Levitsky*, *Division of Nutritional Sciences, Cornell University, Ithaca, New York, 14853–6301, USA*

S. A. Richardson, *Department of Pediatrics, Albert Einstein College of Medicine, 1300 Morris Park Avenue, Bronx, New York 10461, USA*

L. Sinisterra, *Fundacion de Investigaciones de Ecologia Humana, Apartado Aéreo 7308, Cali, Colombia*

J. L. Smart, *Department of Child Health, The Medical School, Oxford Road, Manchester M13 9PT UK.*

*Not present for the Workshop Discussions.

Contents

Preface

During the first quarter of the twentieth century there was considerable interest, in nutritional and other research circles, in the possibility that undernutrition in early life might interfere with the proper development of the brain, and hence might affect the later achievement of the individual. Perhaps, in this post-Victorian era, many research scientists lived fairly close to social underprivilege and would themselves have witnessed childhood poverty in their societies, much as we, today, "witness" it on our television screens in almost daily reports from impoverished communities throughout the world. In both cases, in both the first and in the recent third quarter of the century, social and humanitarian concern amongst medical and other scientists has probably been the main driving force motivating their work, as well as their usual scientific curiosity. In the latter period it has quite certainly influenced grant-giving organizations, including politicians, into funding the very many field and laboratory investigations of the question.

Almost all of the research before 1925 was done in the laboratory, using developing rats, and almost all of it demonstrated a virtually total sparing of the brain, compared with the effects of developmental undernutrition on the other organs and on the body as a whole. When it came to adult undernutrition, the most striking finding was that prolonged starvation, even unto death, left the brain quite untouched, not only in its weight, but also in its detailed chemical composition, in so far as it was possible to measure this at the time. Small wonder, then, that the topic was virtually abandoned.

In the late 1950s it was resurrected. This time the stimulus came firstly from persistent findings in several pre-industrial countries that children performed less well, both at school and in formal tests, when they had histories of undernutrition, especially before the age of two. Secondly, and not much later, it was realized by laboratory scientists that the developing brain was far from unaffected by nutritional growth restriction, provided this was applied during the period of its fastest growth, the "brain growth spurt".

vii

The reason the earlier researchers had not noticed this was that, in using developing rats, they had not begun the undernutrition until three weeks of age, the time of weaning, in a species whose brain growth spurt is over by then, having been encompassed by the suckling period, which is in the first three postnatal weeks. Of course the growth of rats was much easier for them to manipulate after weaning, and at this age there was a great deal of bodily growth yet to be accomplished. By contrast, the brain has a much earlier growth spurt, which was therefore missed.

The moment this was realized, and it largely became so because of reasonably simple new techniques of undernourishing suckling rats by varying the litter size and other means, there began a new spate of investigations in our subject, which paralleled the resurgence of field studies.

During the last quarter of the century, a new situation has arisen, in which increasingly precise and rewarding laboratory studies are continuing, especially in the behavioural sciences and in quantitative neurohistology; whilst the field studies are being much less frequently pursued, as the complexity and the imponderable nature of the human condition is becoming increasingly clear. The great contribution of the best field studies has been to show how many more factors in the physical, as well as in the non-physical early deprived environment, also contribute to poorer later achievement. Indeed it is now a very real and unanswered question whether undernutrition *per se* has any separate role in the undoubted intellectual and social failure to thrive of those undernourished in babyhood? The decline in field studies stems, therefore, from the sheer impossibility both of measuring all these other environmental factors, and analysing and expressing their relative power; to say nothing of the enormous labour involved in coming eventually to a blinding statement of the obvious, that people in poverty do less well in later life than those more privileged. However, perhaps these are only personal views (1). Fortunately the influence of environmental poverty or enrichment, with or without undernutrition, can still be, and is still being investigated in the experimental animal, even though some field workers remain obstinately unconvinced of the relevance of animals to human problems.

Our main question, however, is still immensely important, both socially and scientifically. The above historical note necessarily oversimplifies, and there are many who would argue that it unreasonably exaggerates the difficulties.

The purpose of this book is to examine the present position, first in the laboratory and then in society. It is the result of a special kind of Workshop, designed to display and illuminate those areas which are still being discussed and contested. It answers few questions, since most of the important ones are unanswerable in the present state of knowledge, and many are likely to remain so for a long time, if not always.

Eleven of the most important people in the field were asked to take part in an extensive pre-Workshop discussion by correspondence. Six of them wrote substantial papers in their own subject, and all the papers were precirculated to each of the other ten. Everyone was then asked to write a full commentary on each paper, frankly highlighting any disagreements and differences of interpretation; and each commentary was also precirculated.

When we eventually met together in Paris, we had therefore all seen and digested all the papers, and had had time to ponder everyone else's first, considered reactions. By this stage the original authors had often already amended their papers in the light of the commentaries received, and many of the commentaries had also been modified or replied to in writing.

Neither original papers nor first commentaries therefore needed to be given at the Workshop, which became an occasion for pure, almost open-ended discussion. During this stage further amendments were made to the written work, and new commentaries written on aspects not covered so far.

The result should therefore be a considerable advance on the usual "book of a meeting". All the chapters have been peer-reviewed by the ten other leading people in the field, and all their "referee's" reports compiled, refined and published, a procedure almost unknown to even the most reputable scientific journal. Indeed, unlike the rather trivial "discussion" sections of other books, the commentary sections at the end of each chapter are at least as important, and sometimes almost as extensive, as the chapters themselves.

The reader is therefore put to the singular inconvenience of having to make up his own mind on the most important issues. All we have done is to try to assemble the different points of view from some of the best and most informed practitioners and thinkers in the field. No attempt has been made to reach a consensus, which so often results in a feeble low common denominator, since it fails to display what is the life-blood of progress: the important points of disagreement and their nature.

None of this would have been possible without a Sponsor, and we would like to thank the International Children's Centre in Paris for fulfilling that rôle. This French organization, which does so much for children, especially in francophone developing countries, has an indefatigable President in Professor Pierre Royer, who gave us invaluable encouragement throughout. All the enormous work during the run-up period was in the hands of Dr Anne-Marie Masse-Raimbault and Dr M Chauliac of the Centre. Without them the Workshop could not have happened, and we hope they will find some reward and satisfaction in this resulting book.

John Dobbing

1. Dobbing, J. (1985) Infant nutrition and later achievement. *Amer. J. Clin. Nutr.* **41**, 477–484.

Lasting Neuroanatomical Changes Following Undernutrition During Early Life

K. S. BEDI

Department of Anatomy, University of Aberdeen, Marischal College, Aberdeen, UK

Introduction

The crucial importance of adequate nutrition to the optimal growth and development of humans has been recognized for many years. Despite this, it was only relatively recently that it was realized that there are specific "critical" periods during early life when the human body appears to be particularly vulnerable to the ravages of undernutrition and/or malnutrition (1). Individuals most likely to suffer a period of undernutrition, namely young children, are also those whose bodies are least capable of withstanding its effects. This is because many organs and tissues of the body are still relatively immature and could therefore be profoundly, maybe even permanently affected. The organ of special importance is the brain. After all, it is this that determines the character and intelligence of a person. It is also the control centre for the rest of the body.

Research into the effects of undernutrition on the brain has looked at several different aspects. A wide range of techniques has been employed including biochemical, physiological, morphological and behavioural methods

Early Nutrition and Later Achievement
ISBN: 0-12-218855-1

(2–7). The scope of this chapter is to review critically the experiments that have been conducted to investigate the morphological effects on the brain of a period of undernutrition.

Undernutrition of humans is nearly always complicated by other environmental factors such as disease and social and physical deprivation. The people who suffer from a period of undernutrition are also those who have to endure poor education and housing, and other adverse environmental conditions. This, and the fact that suitable "controls" are often not available, make it very difficult to separate from other complicating factors the effects in man of the level of nutrition. In addition, it is virtually impossible to obtain human brain tissue sufficiently well preserved to enable quantitative morphological investigations to be carried out, especially at the ultrastructural level. Therefore much of the research in this field has been carried out by means of controlled animal experiments, most often using the laboratory rat.

As the timing of growth of the body and brain varies from one animal species to the next, care has to be exercised when attempting to extrapolate from animal studies to the human situation (1). In laboratory experiments the timing and duration of a period of undernutrition of two species may be set with respect to birth. However, because of the possible differences among species in the timing of the "brain growth spurt" (8) that period may have quite different morphological effects. This may be so in several respects such as their severity, location or the structural features involved.

Animal Models

Methods exist which allow rats to be undernourished during any given stage, or combination of stages, of their lives i.e. during gestation, suckling, early postweaning (adolescent) or adult life. In order to undernourish rats during their gestation and/or suckling periods in practice it is necessary to undernourish the pregnant or lactating dams. Undernourishing rats after weaning is relatively easy and simply involves restricting the amount of food made available to the rats to some set level below that eaten by well-nourished, age-matched controls.

Rats can either be *under*nourished (as described above) or *mal*nourished by omitting a specific component, usually protein, from the diet. The idea behind this is to mimic the human condition of protein deficiency. However, it has been found that in some cases the effects of human protein deficiency can be relieved by feeding foods such as carbohydrates (9). This is almost certainly due to the high degree of interdependence of dietary constituents (10).

There is no evidence that the two different types of undernutrition can cause differential effects on the growth and development of the brain. It is more likely that the important factor is that both types can cause growth retardation of the animals at a crucial stage of development of the central nervous system (10).

Although it is of importance to determine the immediate effects of any given period of undernutrition, it is of great significance to establish whether any changes are permanent or not. It is possible that some changes are reversible with a suitable nutritional and/or environmental rehabilitation process. Surprisingly there are very few morphological studies reported in the literature which have paid any attention to this possibility.

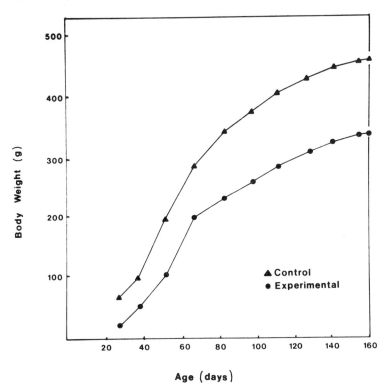

Fig. 1. Body growth curves for control and undernourished rats. In this experiment the rats were undernourished from birth to 30 days of age which resulted in a 70% deficit in body weight. Following nutritional rehabilitation until 160 days of age, the deficit in body weight decreased to about 20%, although in absolute terms the deficit nearly doubled from 50 g to about 100 g. Data from Bedi *et al*. (19).

General Morphological Effects of Undernutrition

Body Weight

Undernutrition of rats during the late gestation and suckling periods causes significant deficits in body weight. Most organs and tissues are affected (11,12). The degree to which any given organ is affected is different for each organ, causing distortions of body structure. Subsequent nutritional rehabilitation of these rats usually does not restore the deficits in body weight.

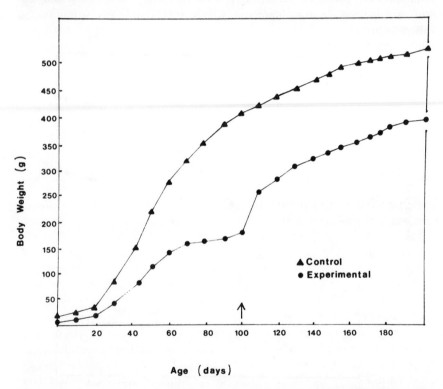

Fig. 2. Body growth curves for control and undernourished rats. In this experiment the rats were undernourished from the 18th day of gestation until 100 days of age, (arrow) after which some rats were nutritionally rehabilitated until 200 days of age. At 100 days of age the undernourished rats has a body weight deficit of about 254 g (59%) compared with age-matched controls. Following nutritional rehabilitation until 200 days of age, this deficit fell to 118 g (23%). In other words it seems that in this instance some "catch-up" growth had taken place during the rehabilitation procedure. Most of this "catch-up" appeared to occur within about 5 days following the end of the period of undernutrition, with very little thereafter. Data from Warren and Bedi (11).

Indeed, it is generally found that although the percentage deficit in body weight of undernourished rats is reduced, the absolute deficit actually increases despite the nutritional rehabilitation. Figures 1 and 2 show the growth curves of control and undernourished rats. In Fig. 1 the rats were undernourished from birth until 30 days of age and then rehabilitated until 160 days of age. In Fig. 2 the rats were undernourished from just before birth until 100 days of age and then rehabilitated until 200 days of age. In both cases it can be seen that the deficits in body weight seem to be permanent. Furthermore, chemical analyses (13) have also revealed that the body composition of rats which have been previously undernourished during early postnatal life is permanently altered. This indicates that the previously undernourished rats are not simply miniature normal rats, but that more subtle changes have occurred.

Not all such experiments reported in the literature (14,15) have shown a permanent deficit in body weight due to undernutrition during early life. The reasons for these apparent contradictions in the literature are not clear. It is therefore of some importance to include full details of feeding regimes adopted and bodily growth curves of animals studied in reports of experiments on the effects of periods of undernutrition.

Brain Weights

Undernutrition of rats during the first half of pregnancy or after weaning causes little or no deficit in brain weight (16). Undernutrition during the latter stages of gestation and the suckling period can cause deficits in brain weight (17–22). These deficits are almost invariably lower in percentage terms than those observed in most other organs of the body. For instance the brain weights for the rats whose bodily growth curves are given in Figures 1 and 2 are shown in Tables 1 and 2 respectively. From these it can be seen that undernutrition from birth to 30 days of age caused "forebrain" (brain minus olfactory lobes, brain stem and cerebellum) and cerebeller weight deficits of about 26% and 33% respectively (Table 1). It is interesting to note that in the second experiment where the period of undernutrition was much longer (i.e. from about birth to 100 days of age), the forebrain and cerebellar weight deficits amounted to about 15% and 20%. In other words, the deficits were smaller in this second experiment than achieved in the first experiment despite the imposition of a longer period of undernutrition.

This demonstrates the high degree of variability which can arise between groups of animals raised at different times. Caution should be exercised when designing and planning such experiments so that the animals in both the control and experimental groups are raised together at the same time, as far as practically possible. Furthermore, close comparisons between results

Table 1. Brain weights of 30- and 160-day-old control and experimental rats.

	Age of rats (days)	Control	Experimental[a]	% Difference
"Forebrain"	30	$1\cdot27\pm0\cdot02$	$0\cdot94\pm0\cdot03^c$	-26
weight (g)	160	$1\cdot69\pm0\cdot05$	$1\cdot46\pm0\cdot03^b$	-14
Cerebellar	30	192 ± 6	129 ± 3^c	-33
weight (mg)	160	300 ± 10	230 ± 10^c	-23

"Forebrain" is here defined as brain minus olfactory lobes, brain stem and cerebellum. Results are mean $\pm$ SE. Data from Bedi et al. (19).
[a] Experimental rats were undernourished from birth to 30 days of age and then nutritionally rehabilitated until 160 days of age. $^b p<0\cdot05$. $^c p<0\cdot01$.

Table 2. Brain weights of control and experimental rats at various ages.

	Age of rats (days)	Control	Experimental[a]	% Difference
"Forebrain"	100	$1\cdot43\pm0\cdot01$	$1\cdot21\pm0\cdot01^c$	-15
weight (g)	200	$1\cdot51\pm0\cdot02$	$1\cdot41\pm0\cdot02^c$	-7
Cerebellar	100	$403\cdot7\pm7\cdot2$	$322\cdot3\pm12\cdot2^b$	-20
weight (mg)	200	$448\cdot0\pm7\cdot6$	$400\cdot0\pm13\cdot6^b$	-11

"Forebrain" is here defined as brain minus olfactory lobes, brain stem and cerebellum. Results are mean $\pm$ SE. Data from Warren and Bedi (11,57).
[a] Experimental rats were undernourished from the 18th day of gestation up to 100 days of age. Some rats were then nutritionally rehabilitated between 100 and 200 days of age. $^b p<0\cdot05$. $^c p<0\cdot01$.

obtained in experiments conducted at widely separate times should only be done with care.

Tables 1 and 2 also demonstrate that the cerebellum was more affected than the forebrain by the periods of undernutrition imposed. This is a common finding in such experiments. It is probably due to the timing of the period of undernutrition with respect to the major phase of cerebellar granule cell development which, in rats, is known to occur during the suckling period (23).

The deficits produced in brain weight by undernutrition during early postnatal life seem to be permanent in most, but not all, studies. Tables 1 and 2 also give the forebrain and cerebellar weight data for nutritionally rehabilitated rats. For these it can be seen that, although reduced by the periods of rehabilitation, the brain weight deficits nevertheless remained statistically significant. Results similar to these have been observed by others (17,24–28).

Some researchers (29,30) have failed to report brain weights of the animals in their experiments. Brain weights provide useful information about the animals under study and give an indication of the degree of undernourishment that has been inflicted on the animals. It is therefore important to report brain weights of control and undernourished animals in any experiments, if this is at all possible.

Effects of Undernutrition on the Microscopic Structure of the Brain

With histological techniques it is first necessary to chemically "fix" all the cellular components of the tissue in a state and spatial arrangement as close as possible to that existing just prior to death. The tissue is then processed for embedding in some medium such as wax, celloidin or resin to facilitate sectioning. The tissue is then sliced into sections. The thickness of these can vary from about 100 μm for some light microscopical techniques, down to about 50 nm for electron microscopy. The sections are normally stained to increase the range of contrast between the various tissue and cell components before being examined with the appropriate microscope.

The processing schedules and the limitations of the microscopical techniques used can all influence the subsequent analysis of the tissue. Many of these important factors have often been disregarded in studies of the effects of undernutrition on brain structure, leaving many of the published results either difficult to interpret, or simply debatable. Some of these results are discussed below in the appropriate sections. First, however, each section begins with an outline of the common errors made in using the various methods, as well as the procedures which can be used to circumvent some of these problems.

Golgi Studies

Golgi techniques can be used to stain a small proportion (between 1 and 3%) of neurons present in a given brain region. The neurons which become stained are usually (but not always) completely impregnated and show their whole extent. The factors governing which neurons actually take up the stain are unknown. It is therefore possible that the stained neurons are unrepresentative of the whole population (31).

Relatively thick (100 μm) histological sections through Golgi stained tissue have been used to trace the dendrites of individual neurons. Even with these thicknesses, it is often not possible to include the whole of a given neuron, including the cell processes, within the section. Golgi stained sections have also been used to quantify a number of features such as dendritic lengths and widths, dendritic branching patterns and the number of dendritic spines per length of dendrite. Dendritic spines are particularly important as they are the sites of at least some, but by no means all, of the synaptic contacts between neurons.

The counts of the number of spines are prone to a number of errors. A major problem is due to the limits of resolution of the light microscopes used to perform such counts. The best theoretical resolution (32) of a conventional light microscope is about $0 \cdot 25 \mu m$. Objectives with a relatively large depth of field, such as those often employed to examine thick Golgi stained sections, generally have a resolution that is substantially worse than this. Dendritic spines smaller than the limit of resolution may not be resolved, and their numbers may be underestimated. Alterations in the size distribution of dendritic spines due to some experimental manipulation can thus yield spurious results concerning the number of spines present per unit length of dendrite.

Another source of error in dendritic spine counts per unit area or length of dendrite arises from the fact that a projected image of the neuron has to be used. "Projection" effects make curved surfaces appear as flat planes. Spines that project at right angles to this plane cannot always be discerned. This can lead to underestimates of spine densities by as much as 20% to 70%. Correction procedures (33) designed to overcome this problem have rarely, if ever, been applied to experimental work on undernourished animals.

A number of studies reported in the literature have examined Golgi stained Purkinje cells from the cerebella of control and undernourished rats. Perhaps the most detailed of these is the study by McConnell and Berry (20,21,26). These workers studied rats undernourished from birth to 10, 15, 20 or 30 days of age, followed in each case by nutritional rehabilitation of at least some animals to 80 days of age. They generally examined the cerebella from ten animals per group. However, from each animal they only examined one Purkinje cell, and thus ignored the within-animal variance. They found that 15 or more days of undernutrition commencing at birth caused significant alterations in dendritic lengths, segment frequency and branching patterns. However, there were no significant differences in spine density between control and undernourished rats. Eighty-day-old rats previously undernourished to 30 days of age showed persisting deficits in overall network size. This was due to a deficit in segment frequency, as segment length did show some recovery. Once again, there were no differences in spine density. Topologic analysis suggested that dendritic remodelling had taken place during the rehabilitation period.

Pysh *et al.* (34) and Noback and Eisenman (27) have confirmed the finding that undernutrition during early life has no significant effect on Purkinje cell dendritic spine density. However, Chowdhury *et al.* (35) have presented contrasting data.

There is also a number of reports in the literature of Golgi-type studies carried out in various neuronal cells of the cerebral cortex. The results presented are not easily comparable with one another, as often different features have been measured. Even in those cases in which the same feature has been measured, the quantitative methods employed and the units used to express the results have varied considerably.

Salas *et al.* (36) have studied rats undernourished for up to 9 days during the first two weeks of postnatal life and found that layer V pyramidal cells had deficits in dendritic density and thickness and spine density. Unfortunately the study was performed on very few animals: two control and three experimental animals per age group. The statistical analysis was questionable as the number of cells examined was used as the sample size instead of the number of animals. This last criticism can also be made of other workers in this field (e.g. 27,37,38).

West and Kemper (37) have studied layer IIb pyramidal neurons of the occipital cortex from rats undernourished from conception to 30 days of age. They reported a deficit in the spine density but no major differences in the total length of basal dendrites in experimental rats.

Leuba and Rabinowicz (39) have studied layers III and V pyramidal neurons from the occipital cortex of control and previously undernourished mice. They found permanent deficits in the extent of dendritic branching and spine density in some (but not all) groups of mice. In general those mice undernourished only during the suckling period showed more permanent deficits than mice undernourished during both the gestational and suckling periods. This is a surprising result and was probably due to the severity rather than the duration of the undernutrition. Mice undernourished during the suckling period alone had a larger body weight deficit than the mice undernourished during both the gestation and suckling periods (39).

It is difficult to summarize the work in the field as there is no consistent theme to the results. This is due partly to the differing periods of undernutrition used and to the different cell types examined in the various studies, but it is also due to the rather unsatisfactory methods used for analysing Golgi stained neurons. In general terms it can be said that undernutrition during early life can cause an alteration in the morphology of Golgi stained neurons with a possible effect on spine density. Nutritional rehabilitation can cause "catch-up" of some features in at least some types of neuron.

Cortical Thickness

Measurements of cortical depths have been used for a long time as a means of quantifying the growth of the cortex. For comparative studies, the method relies on the sampling of accurately matched (i.e. for anatomical location) and orientated (for angle of cutting) sections. Even at best the method only yields fairly crude gross data on the cortical tissue without details about the cellular constituents of cortex, and is thus fairly limited in usefulness.

In one of the first histologic investigations on the effects of undernutrition during early life on rat brain development, Sugita (25) showed that the thickness of the cortex was about 10% greater in underfed animals than in *brain-weight* matched controls. Sugita made no attempt to compare undernourished rats with age-matched controls. More recently, Bass *et al.* (15) have reported substantial deficits of about 22% in the depth of the somatosensory cortex of 10-day-old rats undernourished from birth. However, by 20 days of age this deficit was reduced to about 3%, despite continued undernutrition. Forty- or fifty-day-old rats undernourished from birth until 21 days of age showed no deficits in cortical depths. Unfortunately no statistical analysis of the data is provided by Bass *et al.* (15) and their results must therefore be regarded as rather tentative. A similar criticism can be made concerning data provided by Cragg (40) who reported a 13–15% deficit in the cortical depth of 24- and 50-day-old rats undernourished from about birth.

In a more extensively analysed study, Angulo-Colmenares *et al.* (14) found that 20-day-old rats undernourished from the mid-gestation period had significant deficits in the cortical depths of the somatosensory area. The deficits disappeared following a mere 20 days of nutritional rehabilitation. It therefore seems a fairly common finding that any deficits in cortical thickness produced as a result of undernutrition during early life disappear in later life, at least in rats nutritionally rehabilitated for a short period of time, but thickness, being a linear dimension, is an insensitive indicator of volume, or weight (41).

Neuron Number

Factors affecting counts of neurons

Researchers often claim that they have counted "neuron numbers" in their experiments. Closer examination usually reveals that what has been counted is in fact the numerical density of neurons, e.g. the number of neurons *per microscopic field* or *per unit area of section*. Such counts are not particularly easy to conceptualize. After all, a three-dimensional organ such as the brain does not have an "area" or "microscopic field" as such; it has a volume. It therefore makes more sense to express numerical density data as number of *cells per unit volume of tissue*. Stereological procedures have been derived to enable this to be carried out and are outlined below. First of all, however, it is worth considering the limitations of numerical density estimates and the factors which can influence their determination.

Estimates of numerical density are difficult to interpret, particularly for a developing organ such as the brain (6). This is simply because changes in the numerical density can result from a single factor or a combination of several. Thus changes in the numerical density of neurons can be due to either an actual change in neuron number and/or to changes in the volume of tissue containing the neurons. Estimates of numerical density of various components can, however, be used to calculate useful ratios (e.g. neuron-to-glial cell ratios, granule-to-Purkinje cell ratios, synapse-to-neuron ratios). Such information, which shows the *relative* alterations of two components, are often easier to interpret as they are independent of changes in the volume of the brain.

It would be highly desirable to estimate the total number of neurons within a brain, or brain region, to overcome the problems associated with the interpretation of numerical density estimates. It is tempting to multiply a neuronal numerical density estimate by the volume of the brain and hence derive an estimate for the total number of neurons. However, estimates of numerical density can vary greatly from one brain region to the next, as well as between cortical layers within a region. This heterogeneous nature of the brain makes such estimates of total neuron number quite valueless.

As well as the difficulties associated with interpretation of numerical density estimates, a number of other factors can affect the actual "neuron counts" in histological sections. These are discussed below.

Tissue shrinkage. Histological processing procedures can alter the size of any given brain, usually by shrinkage. This can vary from a few per cent (42,43) for resin embedded tissue, up to as much as 50% for tissue embedded in wax (44,45).

Two types of tissue shrinkage are possible: heterogeneous and homogeneous (46). In the former, various compartments of the tissue shrink at rates different from each other. In homogeneous shrinkage, the degree of shrinkage is uniform in all compartments of the tissue. The problems caused by heterogeneous shrinkage to counts of neuron number are insurmountable. Fortunately such shrinkage can usually be spotted fairly easily as often cells appear "shrunken" into a space smaller than that which they formerly appeared to occupy. Such tissue is usually best discarded from further analysis. Cortical tissue that has been well fixed and embedded shows no such heterogeneous shrinkage.

The problems caused by homogeneous shrinkage are less serious as the degree of shrinkage can sometimes be determined and appropriate corrections applied to cell counts. However, even such shrinkage can cause difficulties in some cases. For instance, it has been found that the degree of shrinkage can be greater in young rats than in older ones (47). It is also possible that the brains from control and experimental animals shrink differentially, despite the careful standardization of experimental procedures. Care has therefore to be taken in the way data is both expressed and interpreted. If the shrinkage within the tissue sampled is homogeneous, then another advantage of calculating and comparing ratios (such as those mentioned above) is that these remain unaffected. This makes it unnecessary to apply correction factors for tissue shrinkage.

Counting unit. The morphological feature(s) used to recognize and count neurons in histological sections can affect the results. Several features have been used as the counting unit for neurons. These include cell bodies, nuclei and nucleoli.

The profiles of most neuronal cell bodies seen in sections are relatively large and easily recognizable structures, and therefore easy to count. These advantages are counterbalanced by the fact that in many cases neuronal cell bodies do not conform to some simple geometrical shape. This can make it necessary to take shape factors (see below) into account when estimating numerical densities using the cell body as the counting unit.

Nucleoli have also been used by some (40,48) as the counting unit for neurons. These have usually been counted in $10-20\,\mu m$ thick Nissl stained sections. It was assumed that all neurons contain a single nucleolus and that glial cells contain none. However, neronal nuclei sometimes contain more than one nucleolus, and it is known that glial cell nuclei also on occasion contain nucleoli. The assumptions are therefore unwarranted. In addition, the relatively small size of the nucleoli (about $2-3\,\mu m$) in relation to the thickness of the sections normally used, make it necessary to focus the section at several different levels through the thickness of the section to perform the counts. The reliability of this procedures is doubtful. Finally the thickness of the section used can itself affect the counts (see below). The nucleolus is therefore not a very satisfactory morphological feature to use for counting neurons.

Neuronal nuclei are fairly easily distinguished from glial cell nuclei and, as the vast majority of mammalian neurons are mononuclear, they have also been used as the counting unit for neurons. The size (diameters range from about $6\,\mu m$ to $12\,\mu m$) and shape (spherical or nearly spherical) of most neuronal nuclei are also convenient in that they pose the least number of problems to the counting and calculation procedures. Nuclei are currently considered to be the most suitable counting unit for neurons (6).

Section thickness. It is reasonably easy to understand that a thick slice cut through an organ containing many particles (e.g. nuclei) is going to contain many more profiles of the particles than a relatively thin slice cut through the same organ. In fact it can be shown mathematically that, for any given size of randomly distributed spherical particles, the number of particle profiles observed in a section is directly related to the thickness of the section. It is therefore necessary to correct for section thickness in any counts performed on histological sections. This factor has been often ignored in studies on the influence of undernutrition on neuronal numerical densities.

Size and shape of particles. Counts of profiles of particles in section can also be influenced by the size and shape of the particles. For instance a highly convoluted and complex shaped particle can, when sectioned, yield several different profiles of varying shape and size (43,49,50), depending on the plane of the section. On the other hand, a spherical particle when sectioned can only yield a single circular profile (43,49,50), irrespective of the plane of the section. It is therefore important to employ particles with a simple and known geometrical shape as the counting unit. Nuclei, the vast majority of which are spherical or nearly spherical, provide such a unit for neurons.

The situation, however, is further complicated because the profile counts are also influenced by the size of the particles (43,49,50). Thus, randomly distributed spherical particles of a large diameter have statistically more chance of being sectioned than those of a relatively small diameter. Once again, this factor has to be taken into account in any estimates of numerical density of neurons (see below).

Stereological methods for estimating numerical density of neurons

Stereology (43,49,50) is the term given to a group of mathematical and statistical procedures which allow the extrapolation of three dimensional structural information from two-dimensional planes taken through the three-dimensional structure. Thin histological sections can be regarded essentially as two-dimensional planes taken through a three-dimensional organ. Stereological methods applied to thin histological sections can therefore be used to obtain quantitative information about the morphological structure of biological tissues.

Stereological methods require that all regions of a particular tissue under study should have an equal chance of being sampled for the counts and measurements. This can usually be achieved by completely random sectioning. However, with CNS tissue this would cause the loss of useful information concerning the spatial arrangement of the tissue. An acceptable compromise is to section the tissue so that the orientation of the plane of sectioning is not random, but its position within the available tissue is random. For instance, cortical tissue can be sectioned such that each section contains the whole depth of the cortex, but the location of the section within the available tissue can nevertheless be kept random. This allows the spatial relationships between neurons in the different layers to be maintained and also gives all portions of the available tissue an equal chance of being sectioned.

The sections produced by this random sampling strategy can then be photographed under a microscope, again using random procedures to select the fields of view (43,49). The micrographs produced are then ready for stereological analysis.

The general stereological formula (50) for estimating the numerical density of particles (e.g. neuronal nuclei) per unit volume of tissue (N_v) is

$$N_v = \frac{N_a}{\bar{H} + t} \tag{1}$$

where N_a = number of particle profiles per unit area of section;
$\bar{H}$ = mean projected height of particles (i.e. the mean height of the particles in all their possible orientations);
t = section thickness.

For spherical particles, the mean projected height ($\bar{H}$) is equal to the mean diameter ($\bar{D}$) of the particles (50).

Estimation of the mean diameter of spherical particles from sectional profile diameters generally requires the application of other stereological procedures, known as "unfolding methods", to the measured size–frequency distribution of the profiles. There are a number of such methods. One of the most frequently used is that described by Saltykov which is quoted and described by Williams (49) and Underwood (50).

It can also be seen from formula (1) that section thickness is required to estimate numerical density. However, if the thickness of the section used is below about 10% of the size of the particles being counted, the errors introduced by ignoring section thickness are negligible. The mean diameters of neuronal nuclei range from about 6 μm to about 12–13 μm. When making counts of neurons it is therefore advisable to use sections with a thickness of about 0·5 μm. Such sections are easily and routinely obtained from resin embedded tissue, which, conveniently, is also suitable for sectioning for electron microscopy. If thicker sections are used, the determination of the exact thickness of each section becomes imperative.

Results

Cerebral cortex. Despite the fact that numerical densities alone are difficult, if not impossible, to interpret, there are a number of studies which have reported such estimates in the cerebral cortex of control and undernourished rats. Many of these studies have not taken advantage of the advances in stereological techniques that were available and have quoted their results in terms of the number of profiles per unit area of section (29,51,52). Other studies (51–53) have used very small numbers of animals or have not carried out appropriate statistical analyses of their results. Some of these papers are discussed further.

Cragg (40) studied 24- or 50-day-old rats undernourished from about birth. However, for each age group he only used one litter from which he obtained four control and four experimental rats. Although it can be advantageous to have littermate pairs as control and experimental animals, it is a disadvantage to have *all* the controls and experimental rats from the same litter. Such a design does not take into account between-litter variance, a potentially important factor in the results.

After killing the rats Cragg (40) used approximately 20 μm thick frozen sections through either the visual or frontal cortices. He used nucleoli as the counting unit to determine the number of neurons per unit volume of tissue. The fact that relatively thick sections were used is probably the greatest source of potential error. It is not considered adequate merely to accept that a microtome set to cut sections at a given thickness will actually do so. In practice sections of a wide range of thicknesses can be produced at any given dial setting on the microtome. The thickness of each section used should therefore be accurately determined, in order to make reliable estimates of numerical density.

Cragg (40) found that the undernourished rats had an increased numerical density of neurons when compared with age-matched controls. Similar observations have been made by many other workers (5,18,28,29,53–55) who have studied rats killed immediately after a period of undernutrition during early postnatal life.

It is of course extremely unlikely that the greater numerical density of neurons could be due to an actual increase in the number of neurons. The phase of neuronal cell production for the majority of the cerebral cortex occurs before birth, and could not therefore have been affected by the postnatal period of undernutrition imposed in the above mentioned experiments. Such undernutrition may however result in a reduced cortical volume due to a retardation of dendritic growth, as observed in Golgi studies discussed above. The reduced cortical volume, together with the possibility that undernutrition of rats during the suckling period does not cause substantial (if any) loss of neurons in the cerebral cortex, would result in an increase in the numerical density of neurons. Unfortunately we cannot be sure, from estimates of numerical density, that undernutrition does not cause the loss of at least some neurons.

It is of some importance to determine whether the increased numerical density of neurons due to undernutrition during early postnatal life is permanent or not. Despite this, few studies have examined this aspect. Some of these are discussed below.

Dobbing *et al.* (51) studied the dentate gyri of two 30-week-old rats which had been undernourished during the suckling period. They found an overall reduction in the neuronal cell densities in the previously undernourished rats compared with controls. This seems to be in contrast with most other studies on neuronal numerical densities. The possible reasons for this conflict remain uncertain as yet but may be due to a combination of some of the possible errors in technique described above.

Siassi and Siassi (28) have also reported some results on numerical densities of neurons in the somatosensory cortex of previously undernourished rats. In one experiment they examined 10- and 21-day-old rats undernourished during gestation. They found that those rats killed at 10 days of age had a 54% greater numerical density of neurons than age-matched controls. By 21 days this difference had disappeared. In another experiment they studied 21-day-old rats which had been undernourished from birth to 10 days of age. Once again rats killed immediately after the period of undernutrition had significantly greater numerical densities of neurons than age-matched controls, whilst rehabilitated rats showed no such differences. Unfortunately the duration of the periods of undernutrition and/or rehabilitation were very short in these experiments. Longer periods could produce quite different results.

Leuba and Rabinowicz (54) estimated the numerical density of neurons in mice undernourished either during the gestation period or the gestation plus suckling periods. The mice were killed at various ages up to 180 days. Mice killed soon after the period of undernutrition had a higher numerical density of neurons than controls. This difference diminished and became non-significant by the end of the period of rehabilitation.

Leuba and Rabinowicz (54) also estimated the volume of the cortex between subcortical landmarks. They used these together with the estimates of neuronal numerical densities to calculate the total number of neurons in the cortex. However, it is difficult to estimate the total number of neurons in the cortex owing to the extremely heterogeneous nature of the distribution of neurons. For example, in Leuba and Rabinowicz's experiments, the numerical density of neurons in the visual cortex of 10-day-old mice varied about twofold between different cortical layers. In addition, there is almost certainly variation between different functional regions of the cortex. It is therefore impossible to determine which value of numerical density to use in estimating total neuron numbers. Taking an average for all cortical regions and layers unjustifiably gives equal weighting to all regions and layers and is therefore unsatisfactory. Leuba and Rabinowicz's (54) results on the effects of undernutrition on total neuron (and glial cell) numbers must therefore be regarded with caution.

Work carried out in my laboratory has shown that undernutrition from birth to 30 days of age results in a greater neuronal numerical density in the frontal cortex than that observed in well-fed, age-matched controls (18). Lengthy nutritional rehabilitation removed any significant differences in the neuronal numerical density between control and previously undernourished rats (19,56).

The question which arises from this observation is whether a longer period of undernutrition starting from around birth and extending into adult life could result in a more permanent change. This question was addressed in a second experiment (55,57) where rats were undernourished from the 18th day of gestation until 100 days of age, some rats being subsequently rehabilitated until 200 days of age. The results obtained in this experiment are shown in Fig. 3. This shows that rats killed during the period of undernutrition had a greater numerical density of neurons than controls at

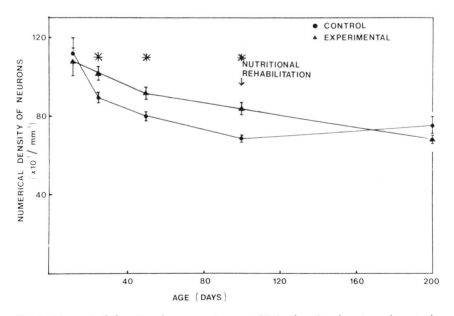

Fig. 3. Numerical density of neurons (mean ± SE) in the visual cortex of control and experimental rats of various ages. The experimental rats were undernourished from the 18th day of gestation until 100 days of age. Some rats were subsequently rehabilitated until 200 days of age. Asterisk denotes significant difference. Data from Warren and Bedi (57).

all ages examined. Two hundred-day-old nutritionally rehabilitated rats showed no such differences. It therefore seems that not even a lengthy period of undernutrition can cause a permanent alteration in the numerical density of neurons. It was also noted that the number of neurons per mm^3 of cortical tissue sampled decreased with age. This is probably due mainly to the increasing cortical volume resulting from an increase in dendritic arborization with age.

In summary, it appears that undernutrition of rats and mice during early postnatal life can cause substantially greater numerical densities of neurons in the cerebral cortex. These increases are probably the result of a reduced dendritic growth, although neuron loss cannot be completely excluded. Nutritional rehabilitation, no matter whether it commences in early preweaning or adult life, is capable of removing the significant differences in the neuronal numerical density estimates. This suggests that perhaps cortical neurons retain their ability for dendritic growth well into adult life. Such dendritic growth would tend to increase the volume of the cortex, which in turn would tend to reduce the numerical density of neurons in the previously undernourished animals to the values observed in controls.

Cerebellar cortex. The cerebellar cortex contains several types of neuron, two of the most easily distinguished of which are granule cells and Purkinje cells. In the rat most granule cells develop postnatally and Purkinje cells develop prenatally. Because of this difference in the timing of development, these cells provide useful indices of the effects of pre- and/or postnatal undernutrition on neuronal development.

Some researchers (20,58) have found that rats killed immediately following a period of undernutrition during early postnatal life had an increased numerical density of granule cells. Others (59,60) have been unable to find any such differences. The exact reasons for these discrepancies remain unknown. However, it seems to be a general finding that nutritionally rehabilitated rats have no difference in the granule cells' numerical density compared with control animals (21,26,60–63).

The observation that undernutrition does not cause a greater numerical density of granule cells than that observed in controls, paradoxically suggests that it may cause a deficit in total number of granule cells. Such a deficit of these cells would tend to produce a lower numerical density. However, if this was accompanied by a reduction in the dendritic arborization of the remaining cells, there would also be a tendency for an increase in the granule cell numerical density. These two separate effects would therefore tend to cancel each other out with regard to their influence on numerical density estimates.

Turning now to Purkinje cells, it has generally been found that rats killed immediately after a period of undernutrition during early life have a greater numerical density of these cells than age-matched controls (20,58,59). In some studies this difference disappeared following nutritional rehabilitation (21,26) whilst in others (60) it did not. However, these findings in terms of neuronal numerical density are, as has been explained above, much less easy to interpret than ratios between cell types.

Some researchers have expressed their data in terms of the ratio between granule and Purkinje cells in order to ease the interpretation of results as mentioned above. Dobbing *et al.* (53) found a suggestion that there was a permanent deficit in the granule-to-Purkinje cell ratio in 30-week-old rats undernourished during the suckling period. However, this study was only based on the cerebella from two control and two experimental animals. This precluded any statistical analysis of the results.

In my own laboratory we (60) have found that 30-day-old rats undernourished from birth have a substantial deficit of about 25% in the granule-to-Purkinje cell ratio compared with controls. Furthermore this deficit was permanent; it did not disappear even after a lengthy period of nutritional rehabilitation (Table 3). Similar findings have been reported by McConnell and Berry (20,21,26). They found that rats undernourished from birth to 20 or 30 days of age had significant deficits in the granule-to-Purkinje cell ratio. Rehabilitation from 20 to 80 days did not restore this deficit.

As Purkinje cells arise mainly before birth in the rat, it is unlikely that undernutrition during the suckling period could cause an increase in their number. The deficit in the granule-to-Purkinje cells therefore seems to provide further evidence that undernutrition during early postnatal life actually causes

Table 3. Data on cerebellar granule and Purkinje cells in control and experimental rats.

	Age of rats (days)	Control	Experimental[a]	% Difference
Numerical density of granule cells in whole cortex $\times 10^3$ per mm^3	30	1187 ± 88	1122 ± 70	-5
	160	768 ± 37	780 ± 62	$+2$
Numerical density of Purkinje cells (per mm^3)	30	3082 ± 263	3960 ± 211[b]	$+27$
	160	2329 ± 112	3185 ± 131[b]	$+37$
Granule-to-Purkinje cell ratios	30	395 ± 34	290 ± 27[b]	-27
	160	335 ± 28	250 ± 23[b]	-25

Results are mean $\pm$ SE. Data from Bedi *et al.* (60).
[a] Experimental rats were undernourished from birth to 30 days of age, after which some were nutritionally rehabilitated until 160 days of age. [b] $p < 0.05$.

a net reduction in the number of granule cells. Such a reduction would be expected to be permanent as the period of granule cell production in rats ends at about 25 postnatal days (23). Accepting this hypothesis makes it not too surprising that the deficit in the granule-to-Purkinje cell ratio produced by undernutrition during the suckling period is also permanent.

Glial Cells

The methods used for counting glial cells are identical with those discussed above for neurons. Many of the workers who have estimated glial cell densities have not accounted for the possible errors previously mentioned; the results presented must therefore be viewed with this limitation in mind. In order to make the interpretation of their numerical density data easier, some researchers have combined their data on neurons and glial cells to estimate glial-to-neuron cell ratios.

Dobbing et al. (53) found that 30-week-old rats previously undernourished during the suckling period had a deficit in the glial cell numerical density in some regions of the dentate gyrus. This change, together with those observed in the neuronal numerical density in the same animals, resulted in a greater number of glial cells per neuron in the previously undernourished rats compared with controls. However, the results were based on very few animals which precluded statistical analysis.

Siassi and Siassi (28) examined 10- and 21-day-old rats undernourished from birth to 10 days of age. In the 10-day-old rats they did not observe any effect of undernutrition on glial cell density although there was a deficit in the glial-to-neuron cell ratio. The 21-day-old rehabilitated rats showed no such difference. Although too close a comparison is not possible because of differing periods of undernutrition and rehabilitation used, the results obtained by Siassi and Siassi (28) seem to contradict those presented by Dobbing et al. (53).

Johnson and Yoesle (52) examined the lateral vestibular nucleus of newborn and 28-day-old rats undernourished from conception. They generally found an increased numerical density of glial cells, a result which once again is in contrast to that obtained by Dobbing et al. (53). Unfortunately Johnson and Yoesle (52) do not provide sufficient details concerning the numbers of animals they examined, the histological and quantitative procedures used for the cell counts and the statistical details of the variance of their data. This makes it impossible to assess the possible validity or otherwise of their results.

Sturrock et al. (64) examined the anterior commissure from 19-week-old mice previously undernourished during the suckling period. They used 6 μm thick serial sections to identify each end of the anterior commissure and then sampled 15 sections from within the commissure per animal. They counted all the nuclear profiles within these sections and multiplied this by the total number of sections containing the anterior commissure. This crude total was then corrected by Abercrombie's formula (65) to obtain a corrected total. They found a significant deficit of about 16% in the corrected total number of glial cells in the commissures of the previously undernourished mice. However, Abercrombie's formula is limited in that when comparisons between groups are to be made, it is necessary to ensure that exactly the same unit area of section is sampled for all animals in both control and experimental groups. Failure to do this can give spurious results. The methods used by Sturrock *et al.* (64) do not appear to have taken this factor into account, and their results must therefore be regarded as rather tentative.

Lai *et al.* (66) examined the corpus callosum of rats undernourished from the sixth day of gestation for various periods of time up to 48 postnatal days. However, they only examined two control and two experimental rats in each day group. Using 1 μm thick sections they observed a substantial deficit in the proportion of oligodendroglial cells at 15 and 21 days of age. However, this deficit disappeared in the 30- and 48-day-old animals despite the continuing undernutrition. This is in contrast to the results obtained by Sturrock *et al.* (64) who found a permanent deficit in the oligodendrocyte fraction, despite lengthy nutritional rehabilitation.

Leuba and Rabinowicz (54) studied mice undernourished during the gestation and/or suckling periods. Some mice were rehabilitated from 21 days of age for various periods of time up to 180 days. They used 25 μm thick cresyl violet-stained paraffin sections to estimate the numerical densities and total numbers of glial cells. The methods used to estimate total glial cell numbers were the same as those used for their neuronal counts described above; similar criticisms apply to their counts on glial cells. Leuba and Rabinowicz (54) did not find any significant differences between age-matched control and experimental animals in the glial cell numerical densities. However their estimates of total glial cell number appeared to fluctuate unpredictably between one age group and the next. For instance there were significant deficits in the total glial cell numbers in the undernourished mice at 10 days of age. Sixty-day-old previously undernourished mice showed no such deficits whilst 180-day-old mice did. It is possible that these fluctuations are not due to any biologic effect but are due to the vagaries of the techniques used to estimate total cell numbers.

It is difficult to reach any firm conclusions about the short and long term effects of undernutrition during early life on glial cells. Some workers have found that undernutrition causes no change in the numerical density of glial cells; others have found it to either increase or decrease with respect to control animals. The contradictory nature of the presently published results on glial cells makes further research into this area of some importance.

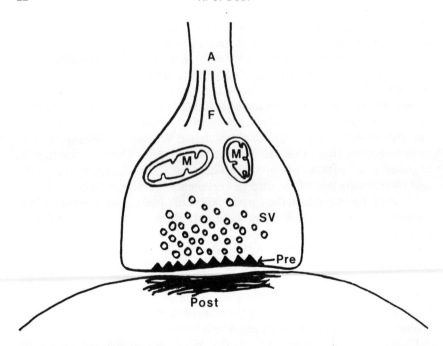

Fig. 4. Diagram to show the general structure of a synapse. A, axon; SV, synaptic vesicles? M, mitochondria; F, neurofilaments; Pre and Post, pre- and post-synaptic membrane thickness (paramembranous densities).

Synapse Morphology

Synapses are points of functional contact between neurons. Electron microscopy has shown that they usually consist of a swelling ("bouton") containing organelles such as membrane bound vesicles ("synaptic vesicles") and mitochondria (Fig. 4). The synaptic vesicles, which contain neurotransmitter substance, are manufactured within the neuronal cell bodies and subsequently transported to the sites of synaptic contact. The actual zone of contact between the neurons at the synaptic sites also has a specialized structure which usually stains densely in nervous tissue processed for electron microscopy. These zones of contact are known as "paramembranous dense zones". The total size of boutons is rarely greater than $0.5\ \mu$m and often they are much smaller. As this is near the limit of resolution of conventional light microscopes, it is necessary to employ electron microscopy to visualise synapses.

Some studies have examined the morphological structure of synapses in control and undernourished animals. For instance, Yu *et al.* (30) examined rats undernourished during early adult life and described unusual lamellar whorls and aggregations of synaptic vesicles. However, Burns *et al*. (67) did not observe any qualitative differences in ethanolic-phosphotungstic acid (E-PTA) stained synaptic junctions from 35-day-old control and undernourished rats.

Jones and Dyson (68) have attempted to quantify the structural components of the synaptic complex in control and undernourished rats. They have measured such things as the lengths of the pre- and postsynaptic membrane thickenings, cleft widths, and the thicknesses of the pre- and postsynaptic dense projections. They have reported that 20-day-old rats undernourished from the ninth day of gestation have deficits in cleft width and the thicknesses of the presynaptic dense projections. The deficits in the latter feature were permanent as they did not disappear, even after lengthy nutritional rehabilitation.

Jones and Dyson (69) have also examined the nature of the curvature of the synaptic zone of apposition. Junctions curved towards the postsynaptic process were designated as negatively curved, and those towards the presynaptic terminal as positively curved. The degree of curvature was represented by letters from A to L, letter A signifying "flat" junctions and B to L representing "increasingly curved junctions". They found that rats undernourished from early gestation till late in postnatal life had fewer negatively curved junctions than at younger ages. The situation for well-fed rats was opposite; they had fewer negatively curved junctions during the early stages of development than at later stages. Unfortunately these studies were carried out on very few animals in any given age group and no information is given as to how many synapses were examined from each. In addition, insufficient statistical details concerning the results are presented making it difficult to assess the validity or otherwise of the data. The biological significance, if any, of the curvature of synaptic junctions remains highly speculative. Certainly there are no strong arguments or evidence to support the postulate by Jones and Dyson (69) that negatively curved junctions are non-functional and that positively curved ones are functional.

Chen and Hillman have reported that 60-day-old rats undernourished from conception have enlarged Purkinje cell spine profiles distributed among normal sized spines. However, they only examined about 90 spines from each of an unknown number of control and undernourished animals and this is insufficient to come to any firm conclusions about the effects of undernutrition on the Purkinje cell spines.

Synapse Number

Factors affecting counts of synapses

As with neurons, researchers sometimes claim to have counted "the number of synapses" in some particular portion of the CNS, when in fact they have made an estimate of the numerical density of synapses. This often turns out to be a count of the number of "synaptic" profiles per unit area of section (35,51,68,71–74). As with neurons, such counts ignore the effects of section thickness and the size and shape of the counting unit used to recognize synapses, and are thus likely to be erroneous. In addition such counts are difficult to conceptualize because, as mentioned previously, biological tissue does not have a "sectional area"; it usually has a three-dimensional structure with a volume.

Three separate morphological features have been used as the counting unit for synapses. These are the bouton (40,75), the total zone of apposition of the pre- and postsynaptic membranes (24,76) and the paramembranous dense zones (18,19,68,77–79). For various reasons the paramembranous dense zone is now considered to be the most satisfactory counting unit for synapses (6,80). It is necessary to assume that these are approximately disc-shaped and that there is only one paramembranous dense zone per "synaptic contact". Serial section studies (81) of synapses have indicated that both these assumptions are reasonable.

Stereological methods for estimating the numerical density of synapses

The general stereological formula for calculating numerical densities of particles on a per unit volume basis has already been given on p.24. It can also be used to estimate the numerical density of paramembranous dense zones (synaptic discs). For disc-shaped particles the mean projected height $(\bar{H})$ is related to the mean diameter $(\bar{D})$ of the discs by the formula (50)

$$\bar{H} = \pi \times \bar{D}/4$$

The mean diameter of the synaptic discs can be estimated from profile size frequency distributions by using identical "unfolding" procedures mentioned above for spherical particles such as neuronal nuclei. Experimental work has shown that the mean diameter of synaptic discs is about 300–350 nm in the rat visual and frontal cortices (19,55).

Results

Many of the results on synapse counts found in the literature have been expressed in terms of the number of profiles per unit area of section and are thus liable to the systematic errors discussed above. A few studies however have expressed data in terms of the number of synapses per unit volume of tissue. Once again it is stressed that numerical density data alone is difficult to interpret.

Cragg (40) was the first research worker to publish estimates of the numerical densities of synapses in the visual and frontal cortices of rats undernourished from birth till either 24 or 50 days of age. In this early work he used the bouton as the counting unit for synapses. The methods he adopted assumed that these boutons were spheres all of the same size, assumptions which are now known to be invalid for most cortical tissue. He did not observe any significant differences in the numerical densities of synapses between control and undernourished rats.

Gambetti *et al.* (51) examined 24-day-old rats undernourished from the late gestation period. They reported small but significant deficits in the numerical density of "presynaptic endings" in the somatosensory cortex of under-nourished rats. Although they studied tissue from four undernourished and three control rats, their statistical analysis was based on the number of blocks used in each group. This artificially and unjustifiably increased the sample size in their statistical analysis, which must therefore be regarded with some caution.

Dyson and Jones (71) have examined the occipital cortex of 20-day-old rats undernourished from conception. They counted the number of E-PTA stained synaptic junctions per unit sectional area and reported a significant deficit in undernourished rats compared to well-fed controls. As well as the possible errors introduced by expressing results on a per unit area of section basis, it seems that Dyson and Jones (71) have also used the number of blocks as the sample size instead of the number of animals. They only used two control and two undernourished animals in their study. Once again, this makes their results and statistical analysis unreliable.

In the same paper Dyson and Jones (71) also report the results obtained from a single 16-week-old rat that had been previously undernourished from conception till 35 days of age. There was no apparent difference in the numerical density of synapses between this and an age-matched control rat. However, no firm conclusions can be reached from this study because of the inadequate number of animals examined.

Similar criticisms apply to a later study by the same researchers (69). In this they examined the molecular layer of the occipital cortex from three sets of rats. In the first set, rats were undernourished from day 9 of gestation to 15, 20, 28, 56, 75 or 224 days of age. In the second set, rats were undernourished to 28 days and then rehabilitated to 224 days. In the third set, rats were fed normally to 28 days but then undernourished to 75 days, when they were killed. However, each age group only contained about two rats which is much too low a number to yield statistically reliable results. Fifteen- and 20-day-old undernourished rats had deficits in the numerical density of synapses. However, 28-, 56-, 75- and 224-day-old undernourished rats tended to have a greater numerical density of synapses than age-matched controls. In the 224-day-old rats previously undernourished to 28 days there were also greater numerical densities of synapses than in controls. Rats undernourished after weaning (i.e. from 28 to 75 days of age) showed no such significant differences from age-matched controls.

In my own laboratory we (18,19,56) found that 30-day-old rats undernourished from birth had significant deficits in the numerical density of synapses in the frontal cortex and granular layer of the cerebellar cortex, compared to well-fed controls. However, these deficits disappeared in previously undernourished rats which had been nutritionally rehabilitated between 30 and 160 days of age.

In a subsequent study (55,57) we examined the visual cortex of rats undernourished from about birth to 100 days, followed in some cases by rehabilitation to 200 days. In this instance we did not observe any significant deficits in the numerical density of synapses either before or after rehabilitation (see Fig. 5).

Synapse-to-Neuron Ratios

When estimates of the numerical densities of neurons and synapses have been obtained on a per unit volume of tissue basis, using the same blocks of tissue,

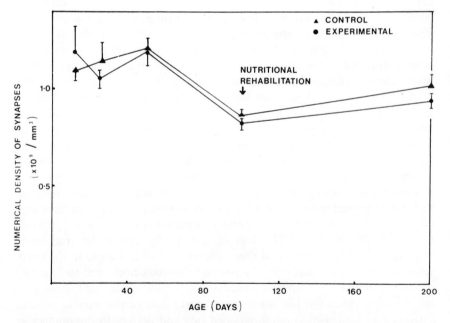

Fig. 5. Numerical density of synapses (mean ± SE) in the visual cortex of control and experimental rats of various ages. The experimental rats were undernourished from the 18th day of gestation until 100 days of age, followed in some cases by nutritional rehabilitation until 200 days of age. Data from Warren and Bedi (57).

it is a relatively simple matter to then calculate the average number of synapses associated with each neuron. As well as being easier to interpret than mere numerical density estimates, it has been suggested (75) that synapse-to-neuron ratios provide a mathematical index of the degree of interconnectivity between neurons. Possible changes in this index due to some experimental manipulation such as undernutrition may provide an insight into the mechanisms of brain development and function.

Despite this, only the studies reported by Cragg (40) and those from my own laboratory have endeavoured to estimate synapse-to-neuron ratios in control and undernourished animals. Unfortunately, Cragg (40) used different pieces of tissue processed in a completely separate way to estimate the numerical density of neurons and synapses. Thus neurons were estimated in frozen sections from one half of the brain and synapses in Araldite embedded tissue from the corresponding region on the other side of the brain.

He found that the frontal cortex of 50-day-old rats undernourished from birth had about 39 800 synapses per neuron. This compared with a value of 60 000 for control rats (see Table 4). The difference was statistically significant. He also observed that in the visual cortex of 24-day-old rats undernourished from birth there were 26 100 synapses per neuron, whereas controls had 38 300. Again the difference was significant (Table 4). Cragg

Table 4. Data on synapse-to-neuron ratios in various brain regions in control and undernourished rats.

	Age of rats (days)	Control	Experimental	% Difference
[a] Visual cortex ($\times 10^3$)	24	$38 \cdot 25 \pm 2 \cdot 82$	$26 \cdot 10 \pm 2 \cdot 91^d$	-32
[a] Frontal cortex ($\times 10^3$)	50	$60 \cdot 13 \pm 4 \cdot 79$	$39 \cdot 83 \pm 1 \cdot 62^e$	-34
[b] Frontal cortex ($\times 10^3$)	30	$22 \cdot 27 \pm 3 \cdot 25$	$14 \cdot 02 \pm 1 \cdot 54^d$	-37
	160	$13 \cdot 36 \pm 1 \cdot 11$	$11 \cdot 80 \pm 0 \cdot 69$	-12
[b] Granular layer of cerebellar cortex	30	495 ± 25	341 ± 17^e	-31
	160	688 ± 38	627 ± 56	-9
[c] Visual cortex ($\times 10^3$)	160	$10 \cdot 29 \pm 0 \cdot 69$	$8 \cdot 99 \pm 0 \cdot 78$	-13

Results are mean $\pm$ SE.
[a] Results from Cragg (40). The rats in this study were undernourished from birth to 24 days of age (visual cortex experiment) or from birth to 50 days of age (frontal cortex experiment)[b] and [c] Results from Bedi et al. (19) and Thomas et al. (56). The rats in these studies were undernourished from birth to 30 days of age, followed in some cases by nutritional rehabilitation until 160 days of age. [d] $p < 0 \cdot 05$. [e] $p < 0 \cdot 01$.

(40) did not investigate whether or not these deficits were permanent following nutritional rehabilitation.

In my laboratory we have now carried out several experiments designed to investigate the effects of different periods of undernutrition followed in some cases by nutritional rehabilitation on the synapse-to-neuron ratios of different brain regions. In the first such study (18) we found that 30-day-old rats undernourished from birth had substantial deficits in this ratio in certain layers of both the frontal and cerebellar cortices (see Table 4). Thus, our results confirmed Cragg's conclusion that undernutrition during early life can cause a deficit in the synapse-to-neuron ratio in certain brain regions. However, there is a considerable discrepancy in the values obtained for the synapse-to-neuron ratio by Cragg (40) and ourselves (see Table 4). For instance, in the frontal cortex we obtained a mean value of about 22 000 synapses per neuron whereas Cragg (40) estimated a value of about 60 000. We believe that this descrepancy is mainly due to the differences in the methodology used by Cragg and ourselves.

Cragg's method of using frozen section for neuron counts and Araldite sections for the synapse counts may introduce several errors of unknown magnitude and sign. In addition, Cragg used nucleoli and axon terminals (i.e. boutons) as the counting units for neurons and synapses respectively. These counting units do not permit the unequivocal recognition of neurons and synapses. For instance, profiles of axon terminals in sections can often be difficult to distinguish from profiles of axons, giving rise to a serious source of potential error.

However, despite these reservations, both Cragg's study (40) and our own (18) showed that undernutrition during early postnatal life caused significant deficits in the synapse-to-neuron ratio. The question therefore arose whether the deficits in the synapse-to-neuron ratio produced by undernutrition during early life persisted into adult life. No previous studies had examined this aspect. We (19,56) found that 160-day-old rats, previously undernourished from birth to 30 days of age, showed no statistically significant differences in the synapse-to-neuron ratio in the layers of the frontal, visual and cerebellar cortices examined (see Table 4).

It was also observed in this study that in the frontal cortex there was a fall in the synapse-to-neuron ratio with age. Thirty-day-old control rats had about 22 000 synapses per neuron whereas 160-day-old control rats had only about 13 000 (Table 4). The fall in this ratio was not as marked in the undernourished animals (Table 4). It was this differential change between control and previously undernourished rats that caused the apparent "catch-up" in the synapse-to-neuron ratio. The falls in the synapse-to-neuron ratio with age were mainly due to decreases in the numerical densities of synapses.

It appears therefore that more synapses are produced in early life than are required in later life, at least in the frontal cortex.

From this study we concluded that the deficits in this ratio, produced as a result of undernutrition during early life, were reversible. Whether this was due to the nutritional rehabilitation or not remained uncertain. It is possible that the "catch-up" in the synapse-to-neuron ratio would have occurred even had the animals continued to be undernourished.

This raised the question whether much longer periods of undernutrition had any additional or more permanent effects on the synapse-to-neuron ratio. This was investigated by undernourishing rats from just before birth till 100 days of age, followed in some cases by nutritional rehabilitation till 200 days of age. In this experiment we (55,57) examined layers II to IV of the visual

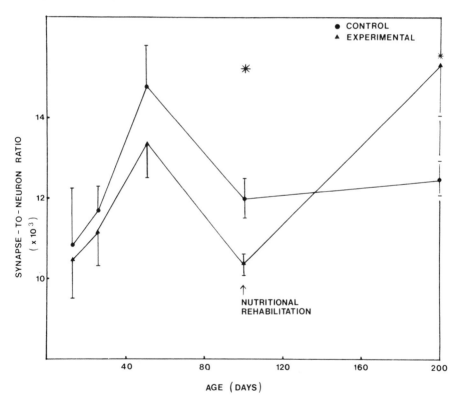

Fig. 6. Growth curves for the synapse-to-neuron ratios (mean ± SE) in the visual cortex of control and experimental rats of various ages. The experimental rats were undernourished from the 18th day of gestation until 100 days of age followed in some cases by nutritional rehabilitation until 200 days of age. Asterisk denotes significant difference. Data from Warren and Bedi (57).

cortex. The estimates of the synapse-to-neuron ratio in this experiment are given in graphical form in Fig. 6.

This shows that, compared to controls, the undernourished rats tended to have a deficit in the synapse-to-neuron ratio at all ages examined up to 100 days of age. The difference reached statistical significance at 100 days of age. However, 200-day-old previously undernourished rats had about 23% more synapses-per-neuron than did controls (Fig. 6). This implies that the previously undernourished rats in this experiment were capable of not only "catching-up" but also overshooting normal values for this ratio. Whether this was due to the nutritional rehabilitation or not remains uncertain.

Figure 6 also reveals that in control rats the synapse-to-neuron ratio increased to a peak at about 50 days of age but then declined to reach a plateau at 100 days of age. This provides further evidence that a greater number of synapses-per-neuron are produced in early life than are required in later life.

The synapse-to-neuron ratio growth curve followed a similar pattern in the undernourished animals until 100 days of age. It was only during the period of nutritional rehabilitation that the pattern became markedly different (Fig. 6). The functional implications of the initial deficit and subsequent "overshoot" in the synapse-to-neuron ratio remain speculative. However, it is possible that *either* a deficit *or* an excess of synapses-per-neuron than normally expected could be detrimental to the animals.

Summary and Concluding Remarks

It seems that undernutrition of rats during early life can cause deficits and distortions of brain structure. Some of these are permanent; others show evidence of recovery in later life. Whether this recovery is due to nutritional rehabilitation or would have occurred despite continuing undernutrition has seldom been investigated, and provides an area ripe for future research.

Both body and brain weights show marked deficits in animals undernourished during early life. Although the brain weight is less affected than other organs and tissues of the body, the deficits in both body and brain weights are permanent; usually they do not recover, even after a lengthy period of nutritional rehabilitation. Within the brain itself some regions seem to be more affected than others. For instance, such a distortion is present when one compares the weight deficits produced in the cerebellum with those in the remainder of the brain. Thus the cerebellum usually shows a more marked deficit in weight than the cerebral hemispheres in rats undernourished during early postnatal life. This is probably due to the timing of a major phase of neuronal cell production in the cerebellum. Most cerebellar granule cell neurons are produced during this early postnatal period.

It is emphasized that great care should be exercised in extrapolating the effects of a given period of undernutrition in animal studies to the human situation. The timing of the brain "growth spurts" in relation to birth can occur at vastly different times in different species (8). For example, a rat's gestational period is three weeks. At birth it has reached a stage of brain growth approximately comparable with a mid-term human fetus. In other words, it is born much less mature than a human baby. By about five days postnatally it has the maturity of a human newborn, a day in the life of a rat being equivalent to about a month in the life of a human at this stage. A rat is usually weaned at about three postnatal weeks of age, by which time it has the maturity of a 2–3 year old human. It reaches sexual maturity at about seven weeks and has a life span of about three years (8). These factors, and similar ones for other species, must be taken into account in any calculated extrapolation from animals to man.

Quantitative neurohistological studies on rats have revealed that undernutrition during early life causes deficits in cortical depths and increases in the numerical densities of neurons and glial cells. These changes do not seem to be permanent, as rehabilitated animals do not show significant differences in these features. Undernutrition also causes alterations in neuron-to-glial cell ratios, but it is uncertain at present whether these are permanent or not. There is considerable evidence to show that undernutrition during early life causes a substantial deficit in the granule-to-Purkinje cell ratio which is permanent.

The heterogeneous distribution of neurons within the brain and the limitations of the quantitative histological methods have made it impossible to estimate reliably total cell numbers. However, there is some limited or circumstantial evidence to indicate that undernutrition during early life can cause a permanent deficit in the total glial cell number and cerebellar granule cell number.

Golgi studies have indicated that undernutrition during early life can cause permanent deficits and alterations in dendritic spines, dendritic network size and branching patterns. However, this does not appear to preclude some remodelling of dendrites during periods of nutritional rehabilitation.

Undernutrition during early life can cause deficits in the numerical densities of synapses and in the synapse-to-neuron ratios. These deficits are not permanent. Some results indicate that previously undernourished rats are capable of "overshooting" the normal values of the ratio obtained from age matched controls. The important factor to note is that this is not "normal" and may therefore in itself be of detriment to the animals. It also seems that the brain makes many more synapses in early life than it requires in later life. Nevertheless, the brain remains sufficiently "plastic" to allow new synaptic contacts to be made between neurons well into adult life.

The functional implications, if any, of these morphological deficits and distortions remain unknown. However, it should be emphasized that, with our present state of knowledge, it is impossible to ascribe a particular morphological alteration to a given change in an animal's behaviour.

Acknowledgements

Financial assistance from the Wellcome Trust, Tenovus, The Royal Society and the Medical Research Council is gratefully acknowledged. I would also like to thank Professor E. J. Clegg and Professor J. Dobbing for their encouragement of my continuing research interests in this field.

References

1. Dobbing, J. (1976). Vulnerable periods in brain growth and somatic growth. *In* "The Biology of Human Fetal Growth" (D. F. Roberts and A. M. Thomas, eds) pp. 137–147. Taylor and Francis, London.
2. Latham, M. C. (1974). Protein-calorie malnutrition in children and its relation to psychological development and behavior. *Physiol. Rev.* **54**, 541–565.
3. Leathwood, P. (1978). Influence of early undernutrition on behavioral development and learning in rodents. *In* "Studies on the Development of Behavior and the Nervous System: Early Influences" (G. Gottlieb, ed.) pp. 187–209. Academic Press, New York and London.
4. Nowak, T. S. and Munro, H. N. (1977). Effects of protein calorie malnutrition on biochemical aspects of brain development. *In* "Nutrition and the Brain" (R. J. Wurtman and J. J. Wurtman, eds) pp. 193–260. Raven, New York.
5. Pollitt, E. and Thomson, C. (1977). Protein–calorie malnutrition and behavior: a view from psychology. *In* "Nutrition and the Brain", Vol. 2, (R. J. Wurtman and J. J. Wurtman, eds) pp. 261–304. Raven, New York.
6. Bedi, K. S. (1984). The effects of undernutrition on brain morphology: a critical review of methods and results. *Curr. Topics Res. Synapses* **2**, 93–163.
7. Bedi, K. S. (1986). Nutrition, environment and brain development. *Sci. Progr.* **70**, 555–570.
8. Dobbing, J. (1981). The later development of the brain and its vulnerability. *In* "Scientific Foundations of Paediatrics", Vol. 2, (J. A. Davis and J. Dobbing, eds) pp. 744–759. Heinemann, London.
9. McLaren, D.S. (1974). The great protein fiasco. *Lancet* **ii**, 93–96.
10. Dobbing, J. (1981). Nutritional growth restriction and the nervous system. *In* "The Molecular Basis of Neuropathology" (R. H. S. Thomson and A. N. Davison, eds) pp. 221–233. Edward Arnold, London.
11. Warren, M. A. and Bedi, K. S. (1985). The effects of a lengthy period of undernutrition on food intake and body and organ growth during rehabilitation. *J. Anat.* **141**, 65–75.
12. Warren, M. A. and Bedi, K. S. (1985). The effects of a lengthy period of undernutrition on the skeletal growth of rats. *J. Anat.* **141**, 53–64.

13. Winick, M. and Noble, A (1966). Cellular response in rats during malnutrition at various ages. *J. Nutr.* **89**, 300–306.
14. Angulo-Colmenares, A. G., Vaughan, D. W. and Hinds, J. W. (1979). Rehabilitation following early malnutrition in the rat: body weight, brain size and cerebral cortex development. *Brain Res.* **169**, 121–138.
15. Bass, N. H., Netsky, M. G. and Young, E (1970). Effect of neonatal malnutrition on developing cerebrum. i. Microchemical and histologic study of cellular differentiation in the rat. *Arch. Neurol.* **23**, 289–302.
16. Zamenhof, S., van Marthens, E. and Gauel, L. (1971). DNA (cell number) and protein in neonatal rat brain: Alteration by timing of maternal dietary protein restriction. *J. Nutr.* **101**, 1265–1270.
17. Smart, J. L., Dobbing, J., Adlard, B. P. F., Lynch, A. and Sands, J. (1973). Vulnerability of developing brain: Relative effects of growth restriction during the fetal and suckling periods on behavior and brain composition of adult rats. *J. Nutr.* **103**, 1327–1338.
18. Thomas, Y. M., Bedi, K. S., Davies, C. A. and Dobbing, J. (1979). A stereological analysis of the neuronal and synaptic content of the frontal and cerebellar cortex of weanling rats undernourished from birth. *Early Human Dev.* **3**, 109–126.
19. Bedi, K. S., Thomas, Y. M., Davies, C. A. and Dobbing, J. (1980). Synapse-to-neuron ratios of the frontal and cerebellar cortex of 30-day-old and adult rats undernourished during early postnatal life. *J. Comp. Neurol.* **193**, 49–56.
20. McConnell, P. and Berry, M. (1978). The effects of undernutrition on Purkinje cell dendritic growth in the rat. *J. Comp. Neurol.* **177**, 159–172.
21. McConnell, P. and Berry, M. (1978). The effects of refeeding after neonatal starvation on Purkinje cell dendritic growth in the rat. *J. Comp. Neurol.* **178**, 759–772.
22. Stewart, C. A. (1918). Weights of various parts of the brain in normal and underfed albino rats at different ages. *J. Comp. Neurol.* **29**, 511–528.
23. Jacobson, M. (1978). "Developmental Neurobiology." Plenum, New York and London.
24. Kemper, T. L., Pasquier, D. A. and Drazen, S. (1978). Effect of low protein diet on the anatomical development of subcortical formations. *Brain Res. Bull.* **3**, 443–450.
25. Sugita, N. (1918). Comparative studies on the growth of the cerebral cortex. VII. On the influence of starvation at an early age upon the development of the cerebral cortex: albino rat. *J. Comp. Neurol.* **29**, 177–240.
26. McConnell, P. and Berry, M. (1981). The effects of refeeding after varying periods of neonatal undernutrition on the morphology of Purkinje cells in the cerebellum of the rat. *J. Comp. Neurol.* **200**, 433–479.
27. Noback, C. R. and Eisenman, L. M. (1981). Some effects of protein-calorie undernutrition on the developing central nervous system of the rat. *Anat. Rec.* **201**, 67–73.
28. Siassi, F. and Siassi, B. (1973). Differential effects of protein-calorie restriction and subsequent repletion on neuronal and nonneuronal components of cerebral cortex in newborn rats. *J. Nutr.* **103**, 1625–1633.
29. Cordero, M. E., Diaz, G. and Araya, J. (1976). Neocortex development during severe malnutrition in the rat. *Am. J. Clin. Nutr.* **29**, 358–365.
30. Yu, M. C., Lee, J. C. and Bakay, L. (1974). The ultrastructure of the rat central nervous system in chronic undernutrition. *Acta Neuropathol.* **30**, 197–210.
31. Smit, G. J. and Colon, E. J. (1969). Quantitative analysis of the cerebral cortex. 1. Aselectivity of the Golgi-Cox staining technique. *Brain Res.* **13**, 485–510.

32. Barer, R. (1959). "Lecture Notes on the Use of the Microscope." Blackwell Scientific, Oxford.
33. Feldman, M. L. and Peters, A. (1979). A technique for estimating total spine numbers on Golgi-impregnated dendrites. *J. Comp. Neurol.* **188**, 527–542.
34. Pysh, J. J., Perkins, R. E. and Beck, L. S. (1979). The effects of postnatal undernutrition on the development of the mouse Purkinje cell dendritic tree. *Brain Res.* **163**, 165–170.
35. Chowdhury, C., Gopinath, G. and Roy, S. (1982). Effect of undernutrition on the maturation of Purkinje cells in the rat. *Ind. J. Med. Res.* **75**, 559–566.
36. Salas, M., Diaz, S. and Nieto, A. (1974). Effects of neonatal food deprivation on cortical spines and dendritic development of the rat. *Brain Res.* **73**, 139–144.
37. West, C. D. and Kemper, T. L. (1976). The effect of a low protein diet on the anatomical development of the rat brain. *Brain Res.* **107**, 221–237.
38. Hammer, R. P. (1981). The influence of pre- and postnatal undernutrition on the developing brain stem reticular core: a quantitative Golgi study. *Dev. Brain Res.* **1**, 191–201.
39. Leuba, G. and Rabinowicz, T. (1979). Long term effects of postnatal under-nutrition and maternal malnutrition on mouse cerebral cortex. II. Evolution of dendritic branchings and spines in the visual region. *Exp. Brain Res.* **37**, 299–308.
40. Cragg, B. G. (1972). The development of cortical synapses during starvation in the rat. *Brain* **95**, 143–150.
41. Dobbing, J. and Sands, J. (1978). Head circumference, biparietal diameter and brain growth in fetal and postnatal life. *Early Human Dev.* **2**, 81–87.
42. Glauert, A. M. and Glauert, R. H. (1958). Araldite as an embedding medium for electron microscopy. *J. Biophys. Biochem. Cytol.* **4**, 191–194.
43. Weibel, E. R. (1969). Stereological principles for morphometry in electron microscope cytology. *Int. Rev. Cytol.* **26**, 235–302.
44. Brizzee, K. R., Vogt, J. and Kharetcho, X. (1964). Postnatal changes in glial neuron index with a comparison of methods of cell enumeration in the white rat. *Prog. Brain Res.* **4**, 136–149.
45. Robins, E., Smith, D. E. and Eydt, K. M. (1956). The quantitative histochemistry of the cerebral cortex. 1. Architectonic distribution of ten chemical constituents in the motor and visual cortices. *J. Neurochem.* **54**, 54–67.
46. Baur, R. (1973). Notes on the use of stereological methods in comparative placentology. *Acta Anat.* **86** (Suppl. 1), 75–102.
47. Mellstrom, A. and Skogland, S. (1969). Quantitative morphological changes in some spinal cord segments during postnatal development. *Acta Physiol. Scand.* Suppl. 331, 3–84.
48. Palkovits, M., Mezey, E., Hámori, J. and Szentágothai, J. (1977). Quantitative histological analysis of the cerebellar nuclei in the cat. I. Numerical data on cells and on synapses. *Exp. Brain Res.* **28**, 189–209.
49. Williams, M. A. (1977). Quantitative methods in biology. *In* "Practical Methods in Electron Microscopy," (A. M. Glauert, ed.). North-Holland, Amsterdam.
50. Underwood, E. E. (1970). "Quantitative Stereology." Addison-Wesley, Reading, Massachussetts.
51. Gembetti, P., Autilio-Gambetti, L., Rizzuto, N., Shafer, B. and Pfaff, L. (1974). Synapses and malnutrition: Quantitative ultrastructural study of rat cerebral cortex. *Exp. Neurol.* **43**, 464–473.

52. Johnson, J. E. and Yoesle, R. A. (1975). The effects of malnutrition on the developing brain stem of the rat: A preliminary experiment using the lateral vestibular nucleus. *Brain Res.* **89**, 170–174.
53. Dobbing, J., Hopewell, J. W. and Lynch, A. (1971). Vulnerability of developing brain. VII. Permanent deficits of neurons in cerebral and cerebellar cortex following early mild undernutrition. *Exp. Neurol.* **32**, 439–447.
54. Leuba, G. and Rabinowicz, T. (1979). Long term effects of postnatal undernutrition and maternal malnutrition on mouse cerebral cortex. I. Cellular densities, cortical volume and total numbers of cells. *Exp. Brain Res.* **37**, 283–298.
55. Warren, M. A. and Bedi, K. S. (1982). Synapse-to-neuron ratios in the visual cortex of adult rats undernourished from about birth until 100 days of age. *J. Comp. Neurol.* **210**, 49–56.
56. Thomas, Y. M., Peeling, A., Bedi, K. S., Davies, C. A. Dobbing, J. (1980). Deficits in synapse-to-neuron ratio due to early undernutrition show evidence of catch up in later life. *Experientia* **3**, 556–557.
57. Warren, M. A. and Bedi, K. S. (1984). A quantitative assessment of the development of synapses and neurons in the visual cortex of control and under-nourished rats. *J. Comp. Neurol.* **227**, 104–108.
58. Neville, H. E. and Chase, H. P. (1971). Undernutrition and cerebellar develop-ment. *Exp. Neurol.* **33**, 485–497.
59. Clos, J., Favre, C., Selme Matrat, M., and Legrand, J. (1976). Effects of undernutrition on cell formation in the rat brain and specially on cellular composition of the cerebellum. *Brain Res.* **123**, 13–26.
60. Bedi, K. S., Hall, R., Davies, C. A. and Dobbing, J. (1980). A stereological analysis of the cerebellar granule and Purkinje cells of 30-day-old and adult rats undernourished during early postnatal life. *J. Comp. Neurol.* **193**, 863–870.
61. Barnes, D. and Altman, J. (1973). Effects of different schedules of early under-nutrition on the preweaning growth of the rat cerebellum. *Exp. Neurol.* **38**, 406–419.
62. Altman, J. and McCrady, B. (1972). The influence of nutrition on neural and behavioral development. IV. Effects of infantile undernutrition on the growth of the cerebellum. *Dev. Psychobiol.* **5**, 111–122.
63. Barnes, D. and Altman, J. (1973). Effects of two levels of gestational lactational undernutrition on the postweaning growth of the rat cerebellum. *Exp. Neurol.* **38**, 420–428.
64. Sturrock, R. R., Smart, J. L. and Dobbing, J. (1976). Effects of undernutrition during the suckling period on growth of the anterior and posterior limbs of the mouse anterior commissure. *Neuropathol. Appl. Neurobiol.* **2**, 411–419.
65. Abercrombie, M. (1946). Estimation of nuclear population from microtome sections. *Anat. Rec.* **94**, 239–247.
66. Lai, M. Lewis, P. D. and Patel, A. J. (1980). Effects of undernutrition on glio-genesis and glial maturation in rat corpus callosum. *J. Comp. Neurol.* **193**, 965–972.
67. Burns, E. M., Richards, J. G. and Kuhn, H. (1975). An ultrastructural investigation of the effects of perinatal malnutrition on E-PTA-stained synaptic junctions. *Experientia* **31**, 1451–1453.
68. Jones, D. G. and Dyson, S. E. (1976). Synaptic junctions in undernourished rat brain—An ultrastructural investigation. *Exp. Neurol.* **51**, 525–535.
69. Jones, D. G. and Dyson, S. E. (1981). The influence of protein restriction, rehabilitation and changing nutritional status on synaptic development: A quantitative study in rat brain. *Brain Res.* **208**, 97–111.

70. Chen, S. and Hillman, D. E. (1980). Giant spines and enlarged synapses induced in Purkinje cells by malnutrition. *Brain Res.* **187**, 487–493.
71. Dyson, S. E. and Jones, D. G. (1976). Some effects of undernutrition on synaptic development — A quantitative ultrastructural study. *Brain Res.* **114**, 365–378.
72. Rebière, M. A. (1973). Aspects quantitatifs de la synaptogenèse dans le cervelet du rat sous-alimenté des la naissance. Comparison avec l'animal rendu hypothyroidien. *C. R. Acad. Sci., Paris* **276**, 2317–2320.
73. Cravioto, H. M., Randt, C. T., Derby, B. M. and Diaz, A. (1976). A quantitative ultrastructural study of synapses in the brains of mice following early life undernutrition. *Brain Res.* **118**, 304–306.
74. Shoemaker, W. J. and Bloom, F. E. (1977). Effect of undernutrition on brain morphology. *In* "Nutrition and the Brain," Vol. 2. (R. J. Wurtman and J. J. Wurtman, eds) Raven, New York.
75. Cragg, B. G. (1967). The density of synapses and neurons in the motor and visual areas of the cerebral cortex. *J. Anat.* **101**, 639–654.
76. Kaiserman-Abramof, I. R. and Peters, A. (1972). Some aspects of the morphology of Betz cells in the cerebral cortex of the cat. *Brain Res.* **43**, 527–547.
77. Cragg, B. G. (1975). The development of synapses in the visual system of the cat. *J. Comp. Neural.* **160**, 147–166.
78. Cragg, B. G. (1975). The density of synapses and neurons in normal, mentally defective and ageing human brains. *Brain* **98**, 81–90.
79. Vrensen, G. and De Groot, D. (1973). Quantitative stereology of synapses: A critical investigation. *Exp. Neurol.* **58**, 25–35.
80. Mayhew, T. M. (1979). Stereological approach to the study of synapse morphometry with particular regard to estimating number in a volume and on a surface. *J. Neurocytol.* **8**, 121–138.
81. Peters, A. and Kaiserman-Abramof, I. R. (1969). The small syramidal neuron of the rat cerebral cortex. The synapses upon dendritic spines. *Z. Zellforsch.* **100**, 487–506.

Commentary

J. Dobbing: Those who are more interested in human field studies of our subject than in the contributions of the experimental laboratory are often quite happy to use what they conceive to be acknowledged anatomical or biochemical "fact" as an alibi for their own interests and beliefs. The laboratory scientist is often just as concerned about human poverty and its consequences, and certainly has just as difficult a task as any field worker. Bedi's paper is very salutary, and should be required reading for anyone (there are many!) who is tempted to display third hand scientific platitudes about "brain cells" and the like in an introduction to his lecture or review. It will be surprising for some, including even some of the best scientists in the laboratory field, to read his strictures on most of the anatomical "findings" in our area.

T. Horwitz: Bedi, in this paper, explicitly restricts his report to "morphological effects on the brain of a period of undernutrition". As a social scientist, i.e. a psychologist, my interest in Bedi's paper directed me to identify those aspects of findings in neuroanatomical studies which would enable me to define observable, if not measurable, behavioural parallels. The central question that emerged in my reading focused on whether it was possible to extrapolate mechanisms or mediating processes leading from the variety of findings with respect to such issues as cell density, cell size, neuron-to-synapse ratios, dendritic arborization, etc., to behaviours which might then lend themselves to psychometric assessment, to systematic, direct observations, and to quantifiable educational and psychosocial phenomena, which could be evaluated in some objective form, etc. This search for mechanisms is, needless to say, a problem which pervades almost the entire effort to discover what the consequences of poor nutrition might be in organic, i.e., anatomic, physiologic, biochemical, or metabolic processes; effects which mediate between the *occurrence* of undernutrition, and *outcomes* in behavioural phenomena including a broad spectrum of such psychological processes as intelligence, cognitive, and social-emotional functions.

At the outset, I was impressed by the multitude of caveats and qualifications which abound in the variety of reports of research which Bedi cites. For example, in many of the investigations described, the number of animals studied is small, or the areas of the brain analysed are limited and circumscribed, or quantitative methods and measures are inadequate or unreliable. Furthermore, undernutrition and the subsequent restoration of normal circumstances when carried out in the animal research laboratory, appear notably different from what occurs in natural circumstances (1), and this also includes in particular the nature of environmental stimulation and social opportunities. Certainly one of the most important issues to consider in this context is the virtually complete reliance in the research studies cited on animal models, particularly the use of the laboratory rat. Nevertheless, despite the obvious shortcomings of this approach, there are significant findings which one must in effect "settle" for from this significant source of data in any effort to establish, even under the most modest "relational premise", the possible significance of such results for the purpose of understanding the human behavioural effects of undernutrition (2).

With these qualifications in mind, let me speculate as to the possible significance of several results which are presented by Bedi. Yet before undertaking this, it is important to emphasize that one must consider the application of results of animal studies to humans within the framework of some theory of human development, in order to justify any effort to assimilate such experimental findings to understanding the effects on a broad array of behavioural entities, including such elusive concepts as "intelligence", "social development" or "cognitive development". In laboratory research with animals the significance of the point at which both the undernutrition and subsequent rehabilitation are introduced become critical, especially when one considers the ambiguous relationship between rat and human life cycles and the existence or lack of existence of corresponding events in the development of the central nervous system in the two species. There are also, in the human organism, other factors which may create areas of disparity with respect to the significance of animal models, such as sex differences in rate of CNS growth in humans, differential rates of maturation and specialization of cortical hemispheres, and maturational processes *within* hemispheres, etc. For example studies of children by EEG methods have indicated a specific vulnerability of the *right* hemisphere to prolonged malnutrition, particularly involving the temporal lobe (3) suggesting that for this reason perhaps "processing of two-dimensional representatives of the three-dimensional world is for some reason below Western standards in malnutrition rife Africa. . .". The lack of cortical specialization in most infrahuman species renders animal findings thus perhaps less meaningful in this context. In any case, the reader is struck by the gaps in our knowledge when one is forced to regard animal studies as a primary or near exclusive source of information on anatomical effects of undernutrition.

An appropriate psychological theory of human development seems essential in considering the potential significance of brain changes as these are related to undernutrition and its subsequent effects on functioning (4–6). Super seems to emphasize a Piagetian approach to such studies as a framework, since it seems more concerned with delineating process rather than reporting the isolated results of purely empirical studies. With this in mind, two findings of morphological changes reported by Bedi are of particular interest in their potential, though speculative application to understanding the possible behavioural significance of early undernutrition in a Piagetian context. In Piaget's theory the early stages of cognitive development emphasize the significant role played by effective motor activity. In this connection, the findings reported by Bedi which indicate that anatomical deficits in the cerebellar areas follow undernutrition may imply deficits which are critical to the development of fine motor coordination and the organism's ability to maintain position in space. Since in Piaget's system, the adequacy of motor development in early stages is crucial for an effective establishment of the entire range of early sensorimotor processes ultimately leading to "object constancy" and to subsequent developmental acquisitions essential for later cognitive maturation, this finding is of great interest. Other studies reported by Bedi (7) have further implicated the rat somatosensory cortex in response to brief periods of undernutrition, even when initial states of *increased* neuron density eventually are restored to equivalency with respect to matched controls. The possible adverse influences of such changes observed in the period of sustained undernutrition are not known, yet the potentially important issue with regard to cerebellar and somatosensory findings may be that these structures are also highly relevant to early behavioural adaptation, and their vulnerability to undernutrition effects may be suggestive with respect to long term neuropsychological and behavioural outcomes. McGuigan's (8) motor reaction time paradigm for assessing undernutrition effects is a model which also emphasizes the integrity of motor behaviour as the basis upon which broader CNS effects of undernutrition may be ascertained, though in this model assessment is through electromyographic investigations. These studies tentatively suggest a possible common ground or connection between the effects of early morphological changes in certain brain structures which are related to later motor and sensorimotor functions.

Additional findings reported by Bedi of interest to the neuropsychologist focus on the effects of undernutrition on the development of the corpus callosum. Studies cited from Lai (9) indicate a transient deficit in this structure in undernourished rats, while Sturrock's (10) results suggest a permanent, rehabilitation-resistant change in the "oligodendrocyte fraction". This would imply that important functions mediated by interhemispheric connections may be, in some fashion, compromised through lengthy periods of undernutrition in early life. Furthermore Bedi's own findings regarding the losses in frontal cortex synaptic density, as well as similar effects in the cerebellum, certainly raise significant possibilities for understanding deficits in behaviour with regard to the quality of later cognitive adaptations, which are dependent upon the integrity of these structures. In this respect I would agree with Dobbing's statement, in his commentary, that "Amongst Bedi's own work, his findings in relations to synapse-to-neuron changes in undernutrition are his most important contribution so far". If in fact this synapse-to-neuron ratio is the "index of the degree of interconnectivity between neurons". It suggests a possible morphological basis for the more sophisticated models of neuropsychological performance as, for example, those described in the approaches of Luria (11), Pribram (12) Teuber (13) and others. One can, though with appropriate qualifications, suggest that Bedi's finding is the possible anatomical basis for deficits in complex cognitive and perceptual intellective adaptations later in life which require extensive "interconnecting". Can it be this that Dobbing refers to when he questions whether a seemingly *temporary* effect, may in fact have long-term implications for later educational success or failure? I would venture to say that such an implication is tenable, and has interesting possibilities for research at a variety of levels ranging from the neurophysiological to purely behavioural studies by psychometric and observational methods. Clearly one must be careful to avoid ill-founded and over-general extrapolations, especially, again, where animal models are concerned, and where such vague concepts as "intelligence" and "development" are central to the definition of dependent variables. Finally, in utilizing animal findings for their significance for the human species it is important to recognize that nature shows a certain profligacy in her treatment of the human brain, i.e. that more cells and more synapses may be available than are necessary, and that the combination of normal "cell death", Hoffer (14), and the capacity for new connections to be formed, give the human central nervous system a special receptivity to rehabilitative experiences, not only in the nutritional realm, but in an interacting relationship to biopsychosocial dimensions as well.

The findings reported in this paper have optimistic implications, i.e. that nutritional rehabilitation can restore at least the morphological deficits to normal or near normal values but what remain unanswered in the final analysis, is that, perhaps with few exceptions, the real source of long range adverse consequences of undernutrition may not simply be the effects of this nutritional experience alone on the brain, but rather more directly reflect the compounding problems brought on in addition by poor social, economic, familial and cultural influences.

1. Dobbing, J. (1970). Undernutrition and the developing brain. *In* Himwich W., "Developmental Neurobiology" (W. Himwich, ed.). Charles C. Thomas, Springfield, Illinois.
2. Smart, J. L. (1984). Animal models: advantages and limitations. *In* "Malnutrition and Behavior: Critical Assessment of Key Issues" (J. Brožek and B. Schürch, eds). Nestlé Foundation, Lausanne, Switzerland.
3. Bartel, P. R. (1976). Findings of EEG and psychomotor studies on malnourished children. *In* "Malnutrition in Southern Africa" (R. D. Griesel, ed.). University of South Africa, Pretoria.
4. Brozek, J. and Vaes, G. (1961). Experimental investigations on the effects of dietary deficiencies on animal and human behavior. *Vitam. Horm.* **19**, 43–94.
5. Dasen, P. R. (1972). Cross cultural Piagetian research: a summary. *J. Cross Cultural Psychol.* **3**, 23–29.
6. Super, C. M. (1981). Behavioral development in infancy. *In* "Handbook of Cross Cultural Human Development", (R. H. Munroe, R. L. Munroe, B. B. Munroe, and M. Whiting, eds). Garland STPM, New York.
7. Siassi, F. and Siassi, B. (1973). Differential effects of protein–calorie restriction and subsequent repletion on neuronal and non-neuronal components of cerebral cortex in newborn rats. *J. Nutr.* **103**, 1625–1633.
8. McGuigan, F. J. (1979). "Psychophysiological Measurement of Covert Behavior—A Guide for the Laboratory." Lawrence Erlbaum Assoc. Hillsdale, New Jersey.
9. Lai, M. L., Lewis, P. D. and Patel, A. J. (1980). Effects of undernutrition on gliogenesis and glial maturation in rat corpus callosum. *J. Comp. Neurol.* **193**, 965–972.
10. Sturrock, R. R., Smart, J. L. and Dobbing, J. (1976). Effects of undernutrition during the suckling period on growth of the anterior and posterior limbs of the monse anterior commisure. *Neuropathol. Appl. Neurobiol.* **2**, 411–419.

11. Luria, A. (1981). "Higher Cortical Functions in Man." Basic Books, New York.
12. Pribram, K. H. "Languages of the Brain." Prentice-Hall, Englewood Cliffs, New Jersey.
13. Teuber, H. L. (1964). The riddle of frontal lobe function in man. *In* "The Frontal Granular Cortex and Behavior", (J. M. Warren and K. Akert, eds). McGraw-Hill, New York.
14. Hofer, W. (1983). "The Developing Brain." San Francisco.

Author's reply: I have only one comment to make here. This refers to Hurwitz's last paragraph where he says that the findings reported in my paper have "optimistic implications". I regret this interpretation. I do not believe my paper leads to optimism at all. I have tried to be neutral.

J. Dobbing: I was glad to read in Bedi's concluding remarks some account of the rules of proper extrapolation of findings to humans from other animals. These rules are surprisingly seldom obeyed.

Bedi makes a very proper criticism throughout the paper of conclusions being drawn from too few animals. Too few have usually been used because the techniques of quantitative neurohistology are very laborious and authors are to be forgiven for only having counted a few. I wonder how much better (from the statistical point of view) his own figures are?

Author's reply: This is an impossible question to answer. However, my figures, which are based on at least six animals per group, are much more reliable than the majority of quantitative morphological studies hitherto reported in the literature, some of which have only used one or two animals.

J. L. Smart: Bedi does those of us who are not quantitative histologists a great service in his review of neuroanatomical changes following undernutrition with his many trenchant methodological criticisms of past research in this area. He rightly criticises several investigators for using far too few animals. This is usually indefensible, but it seems to me that the use of small numbers of animals per data point may sometimes be virtually unavoidable and, indeed, permissible. I have in mind the sort of study in which changes with age are compared between groups: that is, where there is a developmental series for each group (his ref. 68). In such cases each data point is supported by those before and after it, and, which appropriate analysis of variance, valid conclusions can be drawn.

Author's reply: I believe that there is a "hierarchy" of acceptability for the number of the animals used. One or two animals for each control and experimental group is entirely insufficient.

When each data point is supported by those before and after in a developmental type of study, results are only *slightly* more acceptable as interanimal variance within groups is still unknown. This is particularly important in quantitative morphological studies as interanimal variance is often the major component of variance (see 1) . I may add that such data are only more acceptable if they have been properly analysed by suitable ANOVA techniques, and this has not been done in the study referred to by Smart in his commentary.

1. Gupta, M., Mayhew, T. M., Bedi, K. S., Sharma, A. K. and White, F. H. (1982). Inter-animal variation and its influence on the overall precision of morphometric estimates based on nested sampling designs. *J. Micros.* **131**, 147–154.

J. Dobbing: Amongst Bedi's own work his findings in relation to synapse-to-neuron ratio changes in undernutrition are his most important contribution so far. The constant trend seems to be that developmental undernutrition imposed at the vulnerable time produces very substantial deficits indeed in that parameter, but that there is no detectable deficit in later life.

Three observations: firstly let us assume that the deficit at the time is functionally significant. If so the question arises whether a transient deficit of this large magnitude over a not inconsiderable period of early life (in human terms) may have serious implications for the educative process, using "educative" in its widest sense? To oversimplify, we all know the apparent effects of missing a crucial term at school on our mathematical or linguistic prowess later. Secondly it may be important to stress that it is a failure to demonstrate *statistically significant* deficits later which is the finding. Is it possible that, for example, increasing variance or some other factor, is masking some permanent residual deficit in the small number of animals studied? Even so there is clearly quite a contraction of the deficit. Finally, I have always thought it important to emphasize, for those mainly interested in the human situation, that the term "rehabilitated" when referred to experimental animals means an *ad lib.* supply, for the rest of life, of a highly nutritious diet, and freedom from preventable disease. Comparable circumstances, regrettably, are not commonly found with humans. The more interesting finding in animals may well be those effects which persist with continuing and continuous undernutrition of some degree.

Author's reply: Dobbing asks whether a transient deficit in the synapse-to-neuron ratio could not have some permanent effect on the function of the brain even though the deficit in the synapse-to-neuron ratio may disappear in later life. My answer to this is yes. I would also add that my most recent studies have indicated that the synapse-to-neuron ratio not only "catches-up" but overshoots the values seen in the control animals (see Fig. 6). I think that what is important is that the synapse-to-neuron ratio is not "normal" even in the nutritionally rehabilitated animals and this may of itself be of detriment to the animal.

Another point worth mentioning is that the methods used only give an estimate of the *average* number of synapses associated with each neuron. They do not provide any information on the *qualitative* distribution of the synapses on the neuron. It is quite feasible that there could be an alteration in the distribution of synapses due to undernutrition without there being a change in the average number of synapses-per-neuron. Such qualitative changes could also affect the "functioning" of the brain.

J. L. Smart: Bedi is very cautious in his conclusions regarding total numbers of cells, especially glial cells, mainly because of quantitative histological considerations. He concludes only that ". . . there is some limited or circumstantial evidence to indicate that undernutrition during early life can cause a permanent deficit in the total glial cell number. . ." (p.31). I think that I would conclude that this is highly likely to be so, on the admittedly circumstantial but very persuasive evidence of consistent deficits in total forebrain DNA in adult rats undernourished as sucklings (1,2).

Another point that I should like to make strongly is that, just as some of the behavioural sequelae of early life undernutrition may be attributable to side-effects of the procedures used to produce the undernutrition, so too may be some of the neuroanatomical effects, given that environmental manipulations both before (3,4) and after weaning (5) have been found to result in altered brain structure in the rat. This possibility should always be borne in mind.

1. Dickerson, J. W. T. and McAnulty, P. A. (1972). Effect of undernutrition before and after birth on the growth and development of the rat brain. *Resuscitation* **1**, 61–68.
2. Smart, J. L., Dobbing, J., Adlard, B. P. F., Lynch, A. and Sands, J. (1973). Vulnerability of developing brain: relative effects of growth restriction during the fetal and suckling periods on behavior and brain composition of adult rats. *J. Nutr.* **103**, 1327–1338.
3. Altman, J., Das, G. D. and Anderson, N. J. (1968). Effects of infantile handling on morphological development of the rat brain: an exploratory study. *Dev. Psychobiol.* **1**, 10–20.
4. Szeligo, F. and Leblond, C. P. (1977). Response of the three main types of glial cells of cortex and corpus callosum in rats handled during suckling and exposed to enriched, control and impoverished environments following weaning. *J. Comp. Neurol.* **172**, 147–264.
5. Rosenzweig, M. R. and Bennett, E. L. (1977). Effects of environmental enrichment or impoverishment on learning and on brain values in rodents. *In* "Genetics, Environment and Intelligence" (A. Oliverio, ed.) pp. 163–196. North Holland, Amsterdam.

Author's reply: Biochemical measurements of DNA done on the brains of undernourished animals show that there is a deficit in the total number of cells present, but they do not demonstrate that this is due to a deficit of glial cells. Morphological studies have not (so far) been able to demonstrate a deficit in the total number of neurons and/or glial cells. There is no doubt that there is a deficit in the number of cells, but whether this is due to glial and/or neurons remains to be proven.

I am aware that the procedures commonly used to undernourish pre-weanling rats can also affect the mother–pup and pup–pup interactions. This can alter the environment in such a way that it does not resemble that in which the well-fed pups are raised. Additionally I am aware that such an alteration in the environment could cause morphological changes in the brain which could make it difficult to separate the effects of the undernutrition *per se*. I have discussed this point briefly elsewhere (see ref. 6 of my paper) but acknowledge that I should restate this point more clearly and emphatically in future publications.

I also think that we should strive to use methods of undernutrition (e.g. artificial rearing) to try to circumvent this problem in some future studies. However, I also must contend that the evidence that you quote indicating that environmental manipulation both before and after weaning affects brain morphology, is I believe neither strong nor convincing. It can be criticized in many ways. Indeed I have done just this for some of the work you quote in a recent review (1).

1. Bedi, K. S. and Bhide, P. G. (in press). "Effects of Environmental Diversity on Brain Morphology." *In* "Current Topics in Research on Synapses," (D. G. Jones, ed.). A. R. Liss, New York.

Editor's note: *For further discussion of experimental studies of environmental factors, see Commentary on Smart's paper.*

Linda S. Crnic: Bedi makes several very important methodological points: it is striking that investigators have used sophisticated technology to make measurements of the brain and then made simple logical errors which invalidate the interpretation of the data. I would like to extend the sorts of considerations Bedi raises to the area of neurochemistry. There is a very difficult, as yet unresolved, problem involved in the interpretation of effects of malnutrition on neurotransmitters. It is obvious that one cannot measure absolute amounts of neurotransmitters and make any comparisons between undernourished animals and controls because of the differences in the size of the brains. Not so obvious is the fact that expressing neurotransmitter levels per gram of brain is no solution to this problem. As Bedi points out, the evidence of the effects of malnutrition on glial cells is mixed, but from what we know of brain development, we would expect the glia-to-neuron ratio to be altered by malnutrition, most likely for there to be fewer glial cells. Bedi notes that some evidence for this exists in the general finding of increased neuronal density in malnourished rats. Thus, neurotransmitters expressed per gram of brain cannot be comparable between malnourished and control animals. This is just one of the many considerations which make it difficult to interpret measures of neurotransmitter levels (leaving aside the question of the usefulness of neurotransmitter levels versus turnover).

Perhaps the most important point that Bedi makes is that most research on morphological effects of malnutrition has used brains taken during the period of malnutrition and has not determined the extent of recovery possible. In fact, most studies, including his own, that have looked at brains after extensive nutritional rehabilitation, have demonstrated extensive recovery in all parameters measured. Given the extensive recovery and the fact that the functional significance of the morphological changes remains to be established, we must question the functional significance of the residual brain changes. On the surface, it does not seem to be a good thing to have a smaller than normal brain. We must acknowledge, however, that some of the brain's mass is used to control the vegetative and motor functions of the body. Thus, as smaller bodies need smaller brains to run them (1), it is not necessarily disadvantageous to have a smaller brain to match a smaller body. Indeed, it is well established that the size is large in brain proportion to the body in previously malnourished rats.

There is another way in which the "more is better" mentality may lead us astray in our interpretation of the effects of malnutrition upon brain development. There has been much discussion of the effects of malnutrition on hypertrophy and hyperplasia of the brain, but as yet no analysis of the other important process in development: cell death and synapse elimination. In both central sensory systems and peripheral autonomic and muscular systems, neural connections are overproduced in development, followed by loss of superfluous neurons and synapses (reviewed in 2). This process is often described as "pruning", and elimination of extraneous pathways is necessary for proper function.

Interestingly, Bedi's work provides evidence that the decline in the synapse-to-neuron ratio proceeds in parallel in control rats and rats malnourished throughout the first 100 days of life (see his Fig. 6). As the maintenance of synapses is postulated to involve use of those synapses (2) an interesting question arises as to whether the pattern of synapse elimination is the same in the malnourished as in the control rats. This is a possible neuroanatomical level at which interaction between nutritional and environmental effects might occur.

Bedi presents several extremely important caveats related to the methodology and interpretation of brain morphological studies. This might lead the reader to be discouraged about the prospects for meaningful morphological studies of the brain. However, recent and future progress in the neurosciences has much to contribute to the study of the effects of malnutrition upon the brain, and will no doubt lead to answers to questions of the functional significance of morphological changes. We might anticipate that future progress in computer imaging techniques might increase the efficiency of data collection, and thus allow more subjects to be studied. These techniques might also be used to reconstruct three-dimensional morphology in Golgi studies from the measurement of serial sections and thus help correct the errors due to the two-dimensional nature of brain sections. At present it is an extremely laborious undertaking to reconstruct a single Purkinje cell. Second, the newer functional imaging techniques such as positron emission scanning may help us to understand the parts of the brain used for various functions, and thus the possible disruption or rearrangement of neuronal functioning due to malnutrition. It is extremely important that nutrition researchers make use of the most current technology.

An additional simple strategy which might help to make sense of the apparently contradictory literature in this field is to be aware of the differences between different areas in the brain, both in their time course of development (and thus susceptibility to the effects of malnutrition) and in their normal structure and function. For example, the evidence on the effects of malnutrition on neuron-to-glial ratio seems very mixed until we consider that each of the studies examined different areas of the brain. Dobbing *et al.*'s (3) finding of decreased density of glia in the dentate gyrus and Sturrock *et al.*'s (4) similar finding in the anterior commissure are not necessarily in disagreement with Johnson and Yoesle's (5) finding of increased density of glia in the lateral vestibular nucleus because the former show extensive growth and migration postnatally, while the lateral vestibular nucleus is relatively complete by birth (6). Thus, as we increase our sophistication in conducting and interpreting research, I am confident that we can obtain meaningful data.

1. Jacobson, M. (1978). "Development Neurobiology," 2nd edition. Plenum, New York.
2. Greenough, W. T. and Wallace, J. E. (1987). Effects of experience on brain development. *Child Dev.*, in press.
3. Dobbing, J., Hopewell, J. W. and Lynch, A. (1971). Vulnerability of developing brain. VII. Permanent deficits of neurons in cerebral and cerebellar cortex following early mild undernutrition. *Exp. Neurol.* **32**, 439–447.
4. Sturrock, R. R., Smart, J. L. and Dobbing, J. (1976). Effects of undernutrition during the suckling period on growth of the anterior and posterior limbs of the mouse anterior commissure. *Neuropathol. Appl. Neurobiol.* **2**, 411–419.

5. Johnson, J. E. and Yoesle, R. A. (1975). The effects of malnutrition on the developing brain stem of the rat: a preliminary experiment using the lateral vestibular nucleus. *Brain Res.* **89**, 170–174.
6. Ito, M. (1984). "The Cerebellum and Neural Control." Raven, New York.

D. A. Levitsky and Barbara J. Strupp: We would like to ask whether brain tissue from malnourished or previously malnourished animals is affected by the various staining techniques differently from tissue from well-nourished control animals. Both lipid content and composition, as well as the water content of the body, are affected by malnutrition. Would such changes, or similar ones, result in an error in the interpretation of the anatomical data? If so, are some methods more vulnerable to this kind of error than others?

Author's reply: Any effects on "staining" brought about by undernutrition should only affect quantitative histochemical studies, and not counts of neurons, synapses and glial cells.

L. Sinisterra: Although Bedi often mentions the basic concept of "deficits and distortions", the complementary idea that "there is no lesion" as a consequence of malnutrition during the "growth spurt of brain" should be emphasized.

D. A. Levitsky and Barbara J. Strupp:
Behavioural implications. We would like to comment on the use of neuroanatomical data in the absence of behavioural information as indicators of the lasting effects of malnutrition on behaviour. It is quite possible that malnutrition can produce permanent changes in brain structure without causing any change in brain function (behaviour). For example, one of the major areas of the brain in which early malnutrition produces its most permanent effects is the cerebellum. Yet, we are aware of very few reports of any severe deficits in fine motor coordination, or any other indicator of cerebellar dysfunction, as a consequence of early malnutrition in either humans or animals.

We must also add that it is equally likely that traumatic effects early in the life of a child may have permanent effects on the behaviour of a child without causing any detectable change in brain structure. Although it may be argued that if a change in behaviour exists, so must a change in brain structure; in this case, the psychologist or psychiatrist would have a far easier time detecting the effect of the early experience than the neuroanatomist. But by working together with the behaviourist, the neuroanatomist may have a better chance of finding where in the haystack the small changes in neural structures may lie. It is only when these the two disciplines work together, along with the neurochemists and other neuroscientists, that any significant progress can be made in our understanding of brain structure and brain function and the mechanisms underlying the subtle relationship between manipulation and behaviour.

Sally Grantham-McGregor: It is refreshing to see the problems in techniques as well as the inconsistencies in findings outlined so truthfully. I was under the misunderstanding that measurements in the laboratory were much more "respectable" than those in human field studies. After reading this, I realize we all have our problems!

I was disappointed that neither Bedi nor Smart discussed in any detail studies whereby the quality of the environment is manipulated along with nutritional deprivation. This is an area where animal work could be most useful. In the light of our present knowledge, studies which do not take this into account are unlikely to be relevant to the human condition.

Author's reply: Please see my reference to Bedi and Bhide (1987) in my reply to Smart, page 44. There are very many animal studies on the effects of the environment on both brain and behaviour, and these are discussed in the above review. See also my Commentary on Grantham-McGregor's paper.

D. E. Barrett: Bedi's discussion of the sampling factors which may threaten the reliability of estimates of "neuron number" was extremely clear and showed the advantage of the neuron density approach (which accounts for the influence of particle size and shape and section thickness) for obtaining information about cellular constituents of tissue. I was surprised to find at the conclusion of the paper Bedi saying that the functional significance of structural deficits and distortions was not at all clear. Why is this? One might simply assume that one could malnourish the animals, compare their behaviours with those of animals who were not malnourished, and then (a) examine the effect of the malnutrition on brain morphology and (b) in correlational analyses, try to predict behaviour outcomes from specific structural characteristics; i.e. in the malnourished group. Is the reason that this cannot be done that the very testing of the animals for behaviour characteristics will influence brain development, as the research of Walsh and Cummins (1) would indicate? If not, what are the impediments to research on the functional significance of structural insults to the brain?

1. Walsh, R. N. and Cummins, R. A. (1976). Neural responses to therapeutic environments. *In* "Environments as Therapy for Brain Dysfunction" (R. N. Walsh and W. T. Greenough, eds). pp. 171–200. Plenum, London.

Author's reply: I must stress that estimates of numerical density alone are difficult if not impossible to interpret. It is better to estimate ratios e.g. Synapse-to-neuron ratio; neuron-to-glial cell ratio. Correlational analyses only show associations between two factors—they do not and cannot indicate cause and effect.

The Need for and the Relevance of Animal Studies of Early Undernutrition

JAMES L. SMART

Department of Child Health, University of Manchester,
The Medical School, Manchester, UK

Introduction

There appears to be a greater need than ever before to justify animal experiments and to explain the relevance of animal studies of early undernutrition. The reasons for this seem to be threefold.

Firstly, in the past couple of years the developed Western World has been made aware as never before through the medium of television of the horror and enormity of malnutrition. The plight of the starving in Ethiopia and the Sudan has been forced upon our consciousness as we sit, replete, in our comfortable living rooms. We have been moved to respond (largely individually, little nationally), shamed perhaps by the direct, abrasive Geldof, with gifts to Band Aid, Live Aid, Sport Aid, etc. Quite obviously these starving people need to be fed—immediately. It is facile to conclude that their present need is food and not research of any kind. And yet the more dispassionate, far-thinking observer might suggest that some research might be no bad thing in order to know better how to give the most effective relief in the future; but even he would be likely to decry animal experiments and

Early Nutrition and Later Achievement
ISBN: 0-12-218855-1

to recommend strongly the study of some of the starving, actually in the famine situation. "There are so many starving people in the world, why study animals?"

The second reason stems from the nature of the subject and its history as a topic for research, which now stretches to some twenty years of fairly intense endeavour documented in several hundreds of published papers. I think that it is a fair judgement to conclude that in that time there has not been one "breakthrough" or "discovery", in the sense that the intelligent layman or even clinician would use those terms, of a significant advance in knowledge which greatly increases our understanding of the effects of undernutrition on the development of brain and behaviour. There have been a number of influential hypotheses, most notably Dobbing's vulnerable period hypothesis of brain development (1), Winick's hyperplasia/hypertrophy hypothesis of organ growth (2) and Levitsky and Barnes' functional isolation hypothesis of behavioural development (3), which have stimulated a great deal of experimentation. For the brain at least, the resulting body of information is a substantial monument to the hypotheses that gave rise to it, but none of it has the dramatic impact of a "breakthrough". Of course, those of us actively involved in the subject know that the reason for this is in the nature of the subject itself, which is diffuse and multifactorial even in the confines of the laboratory. More and more, the talk is of interaction of factors, the interplay of undernutrition with other aspects of the young animal's or child's environment, rather than effects of one factor alone. But, of course, for the lay person the conclusion that animal experimentation has helped demonstrate the complexity of the relationship between undernutrition and the development of brain and behaviour is far from satisfying. Better far to have been able to cite one "breakthrough".

The third reason derives from consideration of "animal rights". In the UK at the moment there are a variety of groups, some more responsible than others, who vociferously defend "animal rights", in general deploring the exploitation of animals by man and in particular the use of animals for experimentation. In practical terms, this has led to a more rigorous implementation of the existing legislation controlling animal experimentation in Britain and to the formulation of the new Animals (Scientific Procedures) Bill, now before Parliament, for stricter control (though far from strict enough to appease the animal rights lobby). More generally, the airing of these issues has provoked thought and debate in the scientific community, and has resulted in the publication by some professional bodies of "guidelines" for the use of experimental animals (for example, *Animal Behaviour* (1986); **34**, 315–318). A usual rationalization is that animal experimentation is justified if it will reduce human suffering or significantly advance knowledge. It is a rationalization in terms of costs and benefits; costs to the animal in suffering, against predicted benefits in improving man's lot or man's understanding. It takes only a little further thought to realize that these considerations must become quantitative. Where the stakes are high in terms of possible benefits for man, a greater amount of animal suffering can be justified than when the pay-off is expected to be trivial (4). But who is to make these value judgements and how; and how does one cope with the argument that apparently trivial, academic, research sometimes throws up findings of far-reaching importance? Will human progress be retarded if that type of avenue of advance is barred?

How does animal experimentation on early malnutrition rest within this nest of considerations? Uneasily, I think, for the sorts of reason already put forward above, that no one experiment is likely to lead in itself to alleviation of the human situation or a major advance in understanding. Rather, one experiment contributes to the shaping and consolidation of a body of knowledge which, hopefully, might have these effects. This seems to me a somewhat sophisticated message and would be difficult to put across to an unsympathetic audience.

In the succeeding pages I shall examine the need for and the relevance of animal studies and I shall attempt to do so, not in a proseletysing fashion, but in a balanced way which allows the expression of reservations and misgivings.

I shall adopt the convention of referring to non-human animals merely as animals. Also, I shall often use the term "previously undernourished", usually of adult animals, meaning now enjoying adequate nutrition but having suffered an episode of undernutrition early in life. Such animals are said to be "nutritionally rehabilitated".

Studies which are Difficult or Impossible in Man

Brain

There could be argument, I suppose, over whether or not it is worthwhile to study the influence of early life undernutrition on the brain at all. At one extreme is the attitude that brain development is intrinsically interesting and worthy of study in its own right, without the need to postulate any explanatory or predictive value that such study might have, and at the other is the "Behaviourist" viewpoint that behaviour can be understood in terms of a set of empirically-derived rules and without the need to regard the brain as anything more than a "black box". I prefer to take the stance that the study of undernutrition and brain development might be helpful in (i) elucidating the mechanisms whereby effects on behaviour are mediated, and (ii) predicting what aspects of behaviour might be affected through judicious comparison with known relationships between brain structure and chemistry and behaviour. I use the word "might" advisedly, since, so far, this approach has not proved very illuminating, perhaps because the effects are multi-facetted and not confined to a single system, region, cell population, or whatever.

There is, in fact, only very limited information available on the effects of undernutrition on human brain. With a, sadly, plentiful supply of post-mortem material from children dying of starvation, one might have expected a substantial body of knowledge on the influence of severe, continuing malnutrition on brain, but this is not so. The brains of such children weigh less, contain fewer cells and less total protein and phospholipids, but little more than that is known (reviewed in 5, 6). Because of problems of gaining access to brain material in reasonable time, only those substances or structures are measured that are relatively stable after death, thus precluding much biochemical estimation and most quantitative histological study. Scientifically, animal studies can be vastly superior. The interval between the death of the animal and removal and processing of the brain can be short and, perhaps more important, constant from one subject to the next. Furthermore, for quantitative histological studies (Bedi, this volume) anaesthetized animals can be killed by perfusion with a "fixative" such that their brains are fixed, as nearly as possible, as they were in life. Very often, also, starving children die, not just from malnutrition, but from malnutrition compounded with infectious disease, such that it is impossible to ascribe any observed effects on brain solely to nutritional inadequacy.

If one's interest is in whether there are permanent effects of early malnutrition on brain, effects which are irrecoverable even in the face of continuing, generous refeeding after the period of early insult, then one is virtually obliged to turn to animal experimentation. To answer this question in man requires a most unlikely set of circumstances: that a number of children should experience malnutrition in early life, and should then enjoy a lengthy period of adequate nutrition before meeting with fatal accidents which leave the head undamaged. All this, plus a similarly unfortunate well-nourished comparison group, plus a highly motivated pathologist on call, is too much to expect. Some very rudimentary measurements can be and have been made on aspects of brain structure in children recovering from malnutrition, by transillumination of the head (providing an indication of the width of the subarachnoid space), by echo encephalography (width of lateral ventricles, 7) and more recently by computerized tomography (8). Brain imaging techniques are improving extremely rapidly and may soon be capable of providing worthwhile information on aspects of structure and even, through the likes of nuclear magnetic resonance scanning, about biochemical activity. At the moment the requisite equipment is enormously costly and is unlikely to be found in areas where undernutrition is endemic. However, it is in the nature of technological advance that today's expensive electronic equipment, looked upon now as a luxury, often becomes tomorrow's affordable, routine, screening tool.

Another type of study, which at present would be totally out of the question except in experimental animals, is that of rates of "turnover" (the cycle of synthesis, breakdown, synthesis, etc.) of particular substances in brain, which necessitates sampling brain tissue at prescribed intervals after chemical interference. For example, turnover of the neurotransmitter 5-HT in the brains of previously undernourished animals has been assessed by injecting rats with a substance that inhibits the 5-HT-degrading enzyme and killing them at intervals afterwards to measure the accumulation of the transmitter (9).

Other Organs and Systems

The ability to respond appropriately to unpleasant stimulation or, more generally, to cope with stressful circumstances, is an enormously important aspect of any animal's existence, be it human or otherwise. To ignore this is to ignore a major facet of life, but to study it, except with the mildest of stressors, is unethical in man. One would have to rely on volunteers and these, by definition, are self-selected and likely to be atypical. Laboratory studies with rodents have proved useful in revealing persistent effects of early-life undernutrition on responsiveness to stressors. There have been several reports of changes in the characteristics of the adreno-cortical stress response in previously undernourished rats (10,11) and mice (12), and also the fascinating finding that previously undernourished rats, unlike their well-fed controls, appear to lack the ability to inhibit adreno-cortical responsiveness (13). These endocrine effects, of course, have behavioural implications, and so it comes as no great surprise to learn that behavioural responsiveness to noxious stimulation is altered in previously undernourished animals, specifically in the direction of greater reactivity. Previously undernourished rats are more responsive to electric foot-shock and to loud noise (14–16), and it may be part of the same syndrome that they show heightened responsiveness when deprived of food or water (17,18) and even that they display greater reactivity in social encounters (19) and elevated levels of activity, when this is measured over long periods (20,21). These sorts of findings, taken together, have sometimes been interpreted as indicating that previously undernourished animals have a lowered threshold of arousal; that is, that they require less stimulation to provoke them to act in a particular way (22). Whether or not these effects are, indeed, part of a syndrome with a common mechanism, they are highly consistently in the direction of greater reactivity and are arguably the most reliable set of behavioural sequelae of early undernutrition in experimental animals. The presence or absence of parallels in the behaviour of formerly malnourished children, and whether it is realistic to expect them, is discussed below (pp. 65–67).

The Possibility of Life-span Research

One clear advantage of using rodents for developmental or gerontological research is that their life-span is compressed into two or three years rather than man's "three score years and ten". Indeed Donaldson (23) remarked that a day in the life of a rat is equivalent to about a month of human existence; though this is undoubtedly an oversimplification, as the equivalence in terms of developmental progress is far from linear. For instance, sexual maturity is attained relatively earlier in the rat than in man (about 1/12 of the way into the rat's life-span compared with about 1/6 in man).

The advantages of using a short-lived species are so obvious that they are not worth labouring here. Suffice it to say that there have been hardly any human studies in which formerly malnourished children have been followed up beyond early adolescence. One of the very few examples is the Dutch famine study, which was the product of a unique set of circumstances both at the time of the famine and some eighteen years later through the routine measuring and testing of young men conscripted into the armed services (24), and another is the twenty year study of marasmic children in South Africa initiated by Stoch and Smythe (8). In contrast, in animal investigations of the lasting effects of early malnutrition follow-up to adulthood is the norm.

Even longer-term research on, for example, nutritional influences on longevity, is only possible in any properly meaningful way using experimental animals. Thus there have been demonstrations of greater longevity in rats reared on chronic undernutrition regimes, associated with delayed onset of age-related diseases (reviewed in 25–27). Interestingly, there has been little investigation of the influence of early nutrition *per se* in this context and the findings thus far are so equivocal (28) that further research in this area, though difficult, would appear to be well worth pursuing.

The study of transgenerational effects of malnutrition is perhaps even more dependent on the use of laboratory animals than life-span research and is discussed in the next section.

"True" Animal Models

The term "animal model" is very often used loosely in the context of early malnutrition research to indicate the use of experimental animals to elucidate in general how and in what way malnutrition may affect the development of brain and behaviour in man (29). A more precise usage is to restrict the term to experiments in which an attempt has been made to mimic some human condition or situation. The most notable attempts which have been made in this field of research are those which have sought to replicate the situation of very many human communities in which malnutrition is endemic generation after generation. The publication in 1959 of the results of one such investigation conducted by Cowley and Griesel (30) in South Africa with rats virtually heralded the modern resurgence of interest in longer-term effects of malnutrition. A second study followed in England using dogs (31), to be superseded in the same laboratory by an epic investigation with rats, pursued through some fifteen generations in London (32,33) before crossing the Atlantic to continue for several further generations in Boston, USA (34).

Important questions have been asked of this type of model: whether the effects are cumulative over generations; whether there are transgenerational effects which persist in spite of nutritional rehabilitation, and for how many generations they persist? Effects, at least on growth, development and reproduction, would appear to be cumulative for the first few generations of malnutrition, but then plateau at a fairly stable level and show little further deterioration in succeeding generations (32,33). The reasons for the plateau are not clear. One possibility is that there was little further change because the level of malnutrition imposed was relatively mild and necessitated no additional adaptation. Another possible reason for the plateau is that it reflects a ceiling effect; that is, that some reproductive process is near a threshold state, beyond which it fails altogether. Those above the threshold reproduce at the plateau level, and those below it do not contribute to the next generation (or to the data on its growth and development). Natural selection and physiological adaptation probably play a part, and, possibly, natural selection *for* physiological adaptation.

It seems to be pretty clear that some of the effects of multigenerational malnutrition or even a few generations of malnutrition require more than one generation of adequate feeding before they are fully overcome. Quite remarkably, body growth bounces back to normal or even super-normal levels in the first or second generation of re-feeding (33,34). However, impaired problem-solving ability seems to be more persistent. Cowley and Griesel (35) fed rats a marginally low protein diet for only two generations, re-fed the F_2 young from 35 days and then tested their well-fed offspring as adults. Such rehabilitated rats performed worse in a Hebb–Williams maze than controls with a continuous ancestry of adequate nutrition. Similarly, visual discrimination performance was found still to be impaired in the second generation rehabilitated descendants of rats malnourished for many generations (33,34) though females recovered better in Galler's study.

It is fascinating to speculate why behavioural effects should persist longer than effects on growth. A clue may perhaps be discerned amongst some of Galler's other findings on the same population of rats, in that female rats rehabilitated for one or two generations, when they themselves became mothers, displayed styles of maternal care which were typical of malnourished mothers (36). Such persistence of abnormal maternal behaviour may contribute to continuing behavioural abnormality in successive generations.

These findings, in their totality, have important implications for social and economic planning.

Control and Simplification

One of the most intractable problems in trying to assess the harmful effects of malnutrition on human development is that of separating the effect of this one factor from that of the various other concomitants of poverty. Poor housing and sanitation, disease, lack of education and social breakdown are often inextricably tangled up with malnutrition. The ways in which the researcher in the field attempts to resolve this complex situation will be discussed below. The role of the animal experimenter in this case is clear: to identify the contribution of single factors, most notably malnutrition. A simplified situation can be created, using animals of known genetic constitution which are selected and ascribed to treatment groups in proper scientific fashion, in which all possible aspects of the environment are kept constant except that under investigation (29). Furthermore, animal experiments, unlike human investigations, can be replicated virtually on demand.

Knowledge of the characteristics of the nutritional insult is much more secure in animal than in human studies. Timing and duration can be known with certainty and the more problematical parameter, severity, can be measured at various stages. This sort of information is hardly ever available for children. Very often the best that is known is the timing and severity of the most acute phase, abstracted from hospital records, and with no indication of duration. A further consideration is the adequacy of nutritional rehabilitation after the period of privation. This is readily ensured in animal experiments, but can only be assumed in the human situation. Indeed, one could argue that, after discharge from hospital or rehabilitation centre, the formerly malnourished child is far from being assured of adequate nutrition even when food or cash supplements are available to the family. Ignorance, incompetence and even neglect often predispose to malnutrition in the first place and are likely to continue to pertain after the child returns home unless steps have been taken to combat them.

The field researcher has various devices for trying to overcome these problems. One is to restrict his field to the occasional cases of undernutrition in the developed, industrialized world, which result from specific diseases or conditions such as cystic fibrosis, pyloric stenosis, ileal atresia and protracted diarrhoea (37–39). From the researcher's point of view, these conditions have the advantage that they are not associated with poverty and, hence, he need not be concerned about the contribution of other negative environmental factors. The period of effective growth restriction, however, is usually circumscribed and relatively short—a few weeks or months at most. The findings that such children usually show little in the way of intellectual sequelae from their early experience (37,38) may be attributable, therefore, to the brevity of the period of nutritional lack in relation to the two-and-a-half years duration of the brain growth spurt in man (40). Another instance of undernutrition in an industrialized community was the unique tragedy of the Dutch Hunger Winter of 1944–45, towards the end of the Second World War, in which certain Dutch cities were subjected to severe food restrictions for six months (24). The period of deprivation, amounting eventually to acute famine, ended abruptly with liberation by the Allied forces. An opportunity for follow-up was provided by the routine measurement and testing of males conscripted into the armed forces some eighteen years later. No lasting effects on psychological performance were found, and the same argument can be applied as above that the period of undernutrition was short enough for complete developmental recovery to occur, given good quality nutritional and environmental input.

In Third World locations, in which most research on human malnutrition is carried out, there are several devices that the investigator can employ to attempt to disentangle the effects of malnutrition from those of other factors. Comparison groups of children are often employed who have no documented history of malnutrition and who are said to be of the same socioeconomic class as the formerly malnourished, "index", children (41,42). "Of the same socioeconomic class" usually means school class-mates or drawn from the same neighbourhood and there should always be doubts about the equivalence. Indeed, aspects of non-equivalence sometimes emerge in the course of more detailed study (42). An apparent way of dealing with this problem is to conduct some sort of correlational analysis, in which independent variables, such as nutritional status, social class, home stimulation index, etc., are correlated with a dependent variable, say IQ (42,43). I realize that as a non-statistician I am stepping where angels fear to tread, but it does seem to me that the whole edifice is rather shaky for a number of reasons.

The first is the problem of ascribing a value to the index of nutritional status. Simplest of all possible strategies is merely to rely on the dichotomy, formerly malnourished or well-nourished, index or comparison group, and to conduct the correlational analysis with this either/or input (42), but it has the obvious disadvantage of being qualitative and not a continuously variable quantitative measure as one would wish to have in such an analysis. A second possibility is to create a nutritional index from anthropometric measurements taken at the time of psychological testing; for example, height and head circumference (43), relying on the assumption that they reflect the child's nutritional history. The problem here, of course, is that everyone acknowledges that this assumption is only partly true and that other factors may well have had an important influence on the measures, most notably genetic constitution and disease. Richardson (44), clearly aware of these problems, brought both of the above strategies to bear in the same study and calculated the relative contributions to IQ of malnutrition (index/comparison), height at the time of testing and a social factor score also taken at around the time of testing. It concerns me that the malnutrition and height factors are almost certainly not independent, but I am not competent to say whether this matters. In another analysis of the same study group, a further refinement was introduced, which was to take account of differing degrees and types of malnutrition through weight-for-height and height-for-age measurements at admission to hospital (45). It seems to me that the finer-grained the analysis can be, the more likely is one to arrive at a true assessment of the strength of any associations. Having said this, there are limits beyond which the data from a retrospective study cannot take one. For instance, it will always be unclear whether hospitalization for clinical malnutrition or anthropometric measurements at that stage are due only to poor nutrition or to a combination of factors. Indeed, aware of these considerations Galler *et al.* (46) write very carefully about the influence, not just of early malnutrition, but of ". . . the early history of malnutrition *and its accompanying conditions at the time of the illness* . . ." (my italics).

One of the statistics that can be calculated in correlational analysis is the proportion of the variance in the dependent variable, say IQ, that can be accounted for by variation in different independent variables like nutrition and social factors. It is a sobering finding that often only a small fraction of observed variance is accounted for by the identified factors. For example, the nutritional and social factor indices compiled by Freeman *et al.* (43) between them explained only 6 to 22% of variation in a composite cognitive score, the exact proportion depending on sex and age of the children. Rarely the proportion of total variation accounted for is considerably higher, as in the study by Richardson (44), in which 46% of the variance in IQ was accounted for by malnutrition in infancy, current height and social background score. This would appear to affirm the benefits of finegrained analysis with the identification and assessment of as many factors as possible.

In a further attempt to separate nutrition from other environmental factors, some studies include a sibling control group, who, in the case of Hertzig *et al.* (41), were the nearest-age brothers of index boys, without a history of severe malnutrition. The theoretical advantage of such a group is that they should have shared the same environment as the index children, but without nutritional privation. Further consideration of this proposition soon leads to the conclusion that this is just too good to be true. The question that demands to be answered is "why that child, and not his brother?". Some possible answers are given by Smart (29). It seems to me that this question is amenable to investigation and could yield extremely important information on what might be called the microecology of malnutrition.

The Study of Mechanisms

The study of mechanisms, or the way in which any factor like undernutrition comes to have its ultimate effect, is very often better achieved through animal experimentation than human study. Indeed, the flow of understanding may well begin with a clinical observation or an association derived from epidemiological study, for which the mechanism may be sought through animal investigation. Quite clearly the advantages of animal experiments for

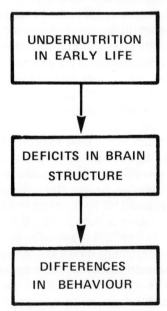

Fig. 1. A possible direct relationship between early undernutrition and behaviour later in life.

elucidating mechanisms are those discussed in the previous section of simplification and of separation of factors.

In the 1960s there appeared to be no need to think beyond the one obvious mechanism. Evidence was accumulating from animal studies of lasting effects of early undernutrition on brain growth (1,2) and the hunt was on for associated abnormalities of behaviour. It was assumed that the relationship shown in Fig. 1 would pertain: that any behavioural impairments were due to deficits in brain growth resulting from the early period of nutritional insufficiency. The period of innocence soon passed as the behavioural studies were handed over by the nutritionists to psychologists and ethologists, who brought with them the new style of thinking about behavioural development that had been evolving in their own disciplines. The new ideas derived largely from animal studies, and I would contend that this extension to the theoretical framework of our subject is one of the major contributions of animal experimentation to research on malnutrition and behaviour, human or animal.

It seems necessary at this stage to put these considerations within the context of the recent history of developmental psychobiology. Freudian theory, that the early experiences in the life of a child leave behind some kind of residue which affects later behaviour, permeated much of the thinking about the ontogeny of behaviour in man and animals in the first half of this century (47). Freud's ideas, of course, derived from clinical observations and not from experimental evidence and, despite their influence on thinking, they were slow to stimulate experimentation; though papers like Hunt's (48) "The effects of infant feeding–frustration upon adult hoarding in the albino rat" were clearly launched out of Freudian theory. However, it was not until the publication of Hebb's book, *The Organization of Behavior* (49), that animal experimentation in this area really took off, encouraged by his plausible postulations regarding the relationship between sensory input in early life and the functional development of the nervous system.

One of the areas of research that grew out of this was that on the effects of early "handling" (or, depending on the experimenter's theoretical orientation, "gentling, stimulation, manipulation, trauma, stress, experience, conditioning", etc.) on various aspects of the development of rodents. Starting with Bernstein (50) and Weininger (51), there followed a stream of papers on the influence of "handling" before or after weaning on survival, maturation, growth, responsiveness to stress, and behaviour (see 52). Usually the effects of handling were either clearly "beneficial" or interpreted as such, including a more adaptive adreno-cortical response to stress. Once the phenomena had been clearly established, the search for mechanisms was soon under way. Much of an insightful chapter by Schaefer (53) is about the quest for a "critical factor", but it is noteworthy in our present context that he entitled the chapter "Some methodological implications of the research on 'early handling' in the rat''. By 1971 some four factors had been proposed, and evidence adduced in their support, which might mediate the effects of early handling, either singly or in combination; namely, direct stimulative action, hypothermia, stress and altered maternal care of the young (54). The last suggestion deserves special attention here because of the influence that it came to have on the interpretation and design of laboratory research in the field of early malnutrition and behaviour.

Ressler (55) addressed the question whether the apparently genetically determined differences in behaviour between inbred strains of mice might be due in some part at least to differences in their postnatal parental environment. His general procedure was to foster-rear two strains of offspring with the same two strains of foster-parents in the four possible strain combinations. He found that offspring of both strains engaged in more visual exploration as adults if they had been reared by one strain of foster-parent rather than the other, and suggested that this might be attributable to the greater amount of handling of the young by parents of that strain. These sorts of considerations were applied to the early handling situation, and soon mothers were found to behave differentially towards treated and non-treated young (56,57). Just how much and in what manner these differences in parental care contribute to subsequent developmental differences has never been satisfactorily demonstrated, but the evidence is highly suggestive of some relationship.

Fraňková (58) was probably the first to incorporate ideas about the undernourished infant animal's environment into her thinking, followed closely by myself and Levitsky. In 1968 she reported the beneficial effects of handling growth-retarded suckling rats on their subsequent behavioural development. In a grant application written in the same year I advocated the use of artificial rearing in undernutrition experiments to obviate the possibility of confounding maternal effects, though it was several years before I put the suggestion into practice (59). The climate then was ripe in 1970 for Plaut's paper (60) on methodological considerations in studies of undernutrition in the young rat, which crystallized the reservations which had been around for a year or two. Basically, the problem is that, in order to have the greatest effect on brain growth, undernutrition is imposed at the time of the brain growth spurt which happens to be when the young animal is still dependent on its mother. Some of the methods of undernutrition during the suckling period quite clearly alter the young animal's environment (Fig. 2). There were soon reports that even the less obviously disruptive techniques resulted in changes in mother–pup interaction (61–64). Despite the considerable ingenuity of researchers in trying to produce a method of undernutrition which would not alter the characteristics of mothering (21,65), I eventually concluded that this was impossible to achieve because of the

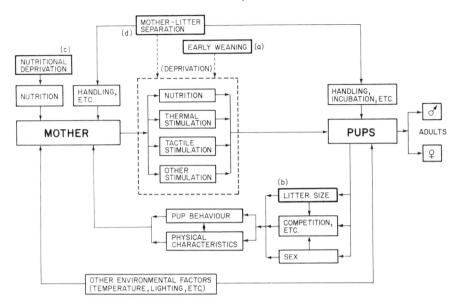

Fig. 2. Plaut's representation of aspects of the mother–litter relationship which may interact to affect offspring development. The letters (a) to (d) indicate different methods of postnatal undernutrition. Reproduced from (60).

obvious differences between well-grown and growth-retarded young. The characteristics of the young determine to a considerable extent the style of mothering they receive and, in particular, small immobile pups elicit more maternal contact than large, active pups (66).

My current view regarding the mechanisms whereby early undernutrition may affect behavioural development is summarized in Fig. 3. It should be noted that although there is evidence, albeit sometimes circumstantial, to support all of the suggested links, there is little indication of their relative strength; that is, of which are the more important. Some would claim that there is only one influential factor, and different individuals might each select a different factor. I incline to the view that it is likely that several factors are responsible for the eventual composite of observed effects, and that this composite of behavioural differences may be due individually to different factors or interactions of factors. Different aspects of behaviour may be influenced through different mechanisms. Furthermore, I do not think that all of the suggested links necessarily have negative effects. Indeed the style of maternal care experienced by undernourished rat pups is highly likely to be of immediate survival value to them and may even result in their behavioural development being buffered from the worst effects of the undernutrition. Additional maternal attention was thought to be beneficial

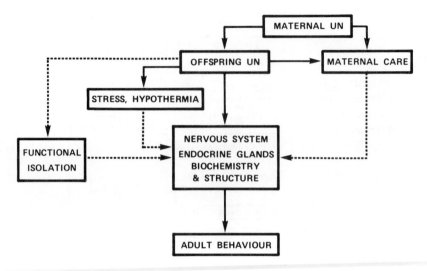

Fig. 3. Possible mediating factors between undernutrition of mother and young and ultimate effects on offspring behaviour. Whether the lines connecting the factors are solid or broken indicates my view of how firm the relationships are: solid, well- or fairly well-established; broken, less well-established.

for Ressler's (55) and Barnett and Burn's (57) mice, why not also for growth-retarded rats?

The situation with respect to mechanisms, therefore, is complicated — even in our simplified animal experiments — and presumably it is orders of magnitude more complex in man. It is probably an important contribution of the animal researcher to have demonstrated not just the complexity of the situation, but the variety and subtlety of the possible influences and the interactions between them. No doubt it would have been more satisfying for the researcher to have been able to prove the existence of a simple, strong relationship, and more comprehensible and acceptable to the layman also; but there is no need to be apologetic. If that is indeed the nature of the situation, then it is valuable to have shown it to be so. It seems quite often to be the case that further study of a subject leads to an appreciation of its greater complexity, as has occurred in the case of diabetes.

Where does all this leave the animal experimenter in the field of early malnutrition and behaviour? Can he still make a worthwhile contribution? It seems to me that useful progress could be made along a number of avenues, only three of which I shall mention here.

(1) A central question remains whether there are lasting effects of early undernutrition on behaviour which are mediated *directly* through restriction of brain growth. It is debatable whether or not this can ever

be answered unequivocally, but two quite different approaches, both unfortunately labour-intensive, ought to take us closer to an answer. One is to employ a variety of quite different methods of undernutrition, presumably with different side-effects, and to assume that if they are found to have a common outcome then that is likely to have been due to the factor of experimental interest, the one common factor, undernutrition (67). The other, which I have chosen to adopt, is to obviate the possibility of confounding maternal effects by removing the mother from the situation altogether and rearing the young artificially (68). Any behavioural differences between previously undernourished artificially-reared and well-fed artificially-reared rats in adulthood ought to be attributable to the growth-restricting effect of undernutrition or to some very close concomitant of it.

(2) A second approach is to investigate other specific possible mechanisms or mechanisms in general. An alternative viewpoint of the results obtained from a variety of undernutrition techniques is not to seek a common effect, as suggested above, but to exploit the occurrence of different effects of different methods (69). Thus a behavioural effect resulting from one method of undernutrition but not another could be attributed to any difference in the indirect effects of the two treatments.

(3) A third strategy is to ignore the issue of whether any effects of undernutrition are directly or indirectly mediated and to study the interaction of other supposedly positive or negative environmental factors with undernutrition. Depending on context the non-nutritional treatment may be imposed before, during or after the period of nutritional restriction. Thus such important questions can be investigated as whether the effects of undernutrition and a second negative factor occurring simultaneously are more or less than additive (70), or whether environmental enrichment subsequent to under-nutrition can have a compensatory effect (71,72).

Cautions

Quite a number of reservations regarding animal experiments have already been expressed in the preceding pages, and so the two categories given prominence below should not be thought of as the only reservations or necessarily the most important ones.

Cross-species Extrapolation

The first point to make is that there are remarkably few species from which to make any extrapolation. The rat has been by far the most popular species.

Eighty-five per cent of all papers on early undernutrition and learning have been on rats, with the remaining 15% distributed between five other species (papers per species: 68 on rat, 7 on mouse, 2 on pig, 1 on cat, 1 on rhesus and 1 on squirrel monkey; ref. 73). To say the least, this is a far from secure basis for any extrapolation from "animals in general" to man.

It is, of course, implicit in any use of animals to elucidate a human condition that there should eventually be some degree of extrapolation. This can usually be accomplished fairly safely and directly at an anatomical and even a physiological level, given the assumption that the mammal under consideration is a sensible choice and not adapted for some extreme environment; but the same cannot be said of extrapolation of conclusions regarding behaviour. The prime reasons for this are man's enormous capacity for learning and his bewilderingly complex behavioural repertoire, both probably associated with the high proportion of "uncommitted" tissue in his large brain and with his uniquely long period of development (discussed further in 29).

Yet within the broad spectrum of behavioural categories there are probably some that are safer for extrapolation between species than others. Certain aspects of emotional behaviour and of learning and memory are likely to be common to most mammals and, therefore, good material for cautious generalization. On the other hand social behaviour can be qualitatively different between species, with communication between individuals sometimes relying on different sensory modalities in different species. Hence, it is probably not surprising that there is no correspondence between the heightened social reactivity of previously undernourished rats (summarized in 19) and the unsociable, withdrawn behaviour of formerly malnourished Jamaican children (74). What is noteworthy, however, is that social behaviour *was affected* in both man and rat. This suggests that different levels of extrapolation might be used for different aspects of behaviour, with tentative prediction of the direction of effects for, say, emotional behaviour, but the suggestion only of some kind of effect for the likes of social behaviour.

There are aspects of the laboratory and field situations which add to the hazards of cross-species extrapolation or at least militate against the likelihood of successfully predicting the direction or uniformity of effects. The environment of the laboratory animal is usually simple, unvarying and unchallenging, whereas that even of a socioeconomically deprived child is relatively complex, socially and materially. The social environments provide a striking comparison. In the laboratory, animals of the same age, sex and nutritional history are usually housed together and may never meet another animal. In contrast, the index child may well interact with all manner of other people with a variety of nutritional and other experience. His development, socially and otherwise, is likely to bear the mark of these influences. The difference in social reactivity of formerly malnourished children and rats noted above may owe much to this sort of consideration. Given the circumstances of index children it is quite likely that some of them will respond with what has been called "learned helplessness" (75); that is, they come to perceive their circumstances as being beyond their powers to influence for the better and give up trying to help themselves, adopting a totally quiescent attitude. Others will see ways of improving their lot and will act appropriately. It may be for these sorts of reason that index children have been classified contrastingly in the same study as more highly active and more lethargic than comparison children (74). As discussed above (pp. 54–55), previously under-nourished rats are usually found to be more responsive and more active, and it may be that index children too have this tendency but that it is overlaid by learned helplessness.

Effects May not be Additive

One tends to think in terms of the various environmental factors that impinge on the young animal having positive or negative effects on its developmental course. It is but a small step further to consider the overall effect of several factors as a sort of algebraic sum of advantage or, more likely, disadvantage. This is a convenient but, of course, an unduly simplistic view of environmental influences on development in many ways. For instance, it is an unwarranted assumption that the effects of two interacting factors should be strictly additive. Indeed, the combined effects of two negative influences such as malnutrition and disease may be appreciably worse than those of either factor alone. An example of this kind of phenomenon, though involving two periods of undernutrition and not a non-nutritional factor, is the synergistic negative effect on brain growth in rats of pre- followed by post-natal undernutrition, the combined effect of which is greater than the sum of the effects of the two periods taken separately (76). One can even imagine a relatively minor factor, perhaps having no harmful effect on its own, interacting with another factor to result in disastrous consequences. Even if early undernutrition were such a "minor" factor—and some would argue that it is—its potential for damage may still be great in interaction with the cluster of negative influences which often pertains in the human situation. As mentioned above (p. 65), the interaction of factors is amenable to investigation using laboratory animals.

Conclusions

Animal experimentation in the field of early malnutrition is probably most clearly necessary for the investigation of effects on brain growth and development, since such research on man can be pursued in only the most rudimentary fashion. Studies of responsiveness to and ability to cope with unpleasant situations is also ethically possible only with animals.

The short life-cycle of laboratory rodents affords the investigator the possibility of life-span research. Studies of undernutrition and longevity and of multigenerational malnutrition can be conducted meaningfully only in such species. Rats with several generations' ancestry of malnutrition have provided a most useful model of one facet of the human situation.

The task of separating the effect of undernutrition from those of other disadvantageous factors becomes possible in the laboratory, where the situation can be greatly simplified through holding all factors constant other than nutrition (and its close concomitants). Such studies and others derived from them provide insight into the ways in which the effects of early undernutrition may be mediated.

Caution is necessary when extrapolating the findings of animal studies to man, especially with respect to certain aspects of behaviour. It is prudent also to bear in mind that the effects of undernutrition assessed on its own as a single factor may be less than when it occurs in association with other negative factors; that is, there may be synergistic effects of interacting environmental influences.

Above all, animal experimentation and human studies should be regarded as complementary to one another. There should be a continuous interplay of ideas, with each approach providing hypotheses for the other to test. The field researcher may ask for controlled animal investigation to substantiate or refine "hunches" derived from field observations. The laboratory worker may suggest on the basis of his experiments that this aspect of behaviour or that possible mechanism may be worthy of study in the field.

Acknowledgements

I wish to thank the Medical Research Council and the National Fund for Research into Crippling Diseases, who for several years have funded the research on early malnutrition conducted by me and by my colleagues.

I should also like to take this opportunity to express my gratitude to Mrs Irene Warrington for her sterling secretarial service to our group over many years. She typed the present paper with great speed and accuracy, and, equally important, with patience and good humour, as she has done so many times before.

References

1. Dobbing, J. (1968). Vulnerable periods in developing brain. *In* "Applied Neuro-chemistry" (A. N. Davison and J. Dobbing, eds) pp. 287–316. Blackwell, Oxford.

2. Winick, M. and Noble, A. (1966). Cellular response in rats during malnutrition at various ages. *J. Nutr.* **89**, 300–306.

3. Levitsky, D. A. and Barnes, R. H. (1972). Nutritional and environmental interactions in the behavioral development of the rat: long-term effects. *Science, N.Y.* **176**, 68–71.

4. Bateson, P. (1986). When to experiment on animals. *New Scientist* **109** (20 February), 30–32.

5. Dodge, P. R., Prensky, A. L. and Feigin, R. D. (1975). *Nutrition and the Developing Nervous System.* Mosby, St. Louis.

6. Chase, H. P. (1976). Undernutrition and growth and development of the human brain. *In* "Malnutrition and Intellectual Development" (J. D. Lloyd-Still, ed.) pp. 13–38. Sciences Group, Littleton, MA.

7. Engsner, G. and Vahlquist, B. (1975). Brain growth in children with protein–energy malnutrition. *In* "Growth and Development of the Brain" (M. A. B. Brazier, ed.) pp. 315–333. Raven Press, New York.

8. Handler, L. C., Stoch, M. B. and Smythe, P. M. (1981). CT brain scans: part of a 20-year developmental study following gross undernutrition in infancy. *Brit. J. Radiol.* **54**, 953–954.

9. Smart, J. L., Tricklebank, M. D., Adlard, B. P. F. and Dobbing, J. (1976). Nutritionally "small-for-dates" rats: their subsequent growth, regional brain 5-hydroxytryptamine turnover and behavior. *Pediat Res.* **10**, 807–811.

10. Adlard, B. P. F. and Smart, J. L. (1972). Adrenocortical function in rats subjected to nutritional deprivation in early life. *J. Endocrinol.* **54**, 99–105.

11. Sara, V. R., King, T. L. and Lazarus, L. (1976). The influence of early nutrition and environmental rearing on brain growth and behaviour. *Experientia* **32**, 1538–1539.

12. Leathwood, P. D. and Bush, M. S. (1975). Avoidance performance and plasma corticosteroid levels in previously undernourished mice. *Prog. Brain Res.* **42**, 209.

13. Wiener, S. G., Robinson, L. and Levine, S. (1983). Influence of perinatal malnutrition on adult physiological and behavioral reactivity in rats. *Physiol. Behav.* **30**, 41–50.

14. Levitsky, D. A. and Barnes, R. H. (1970). Effect of early malnutrition on the reaction of adult rats to aversive stimuli. *Nature, Lond.* **225**, 468–469.

15. Smart, J. L., Whatson, T. S. and Dobbing, J. (1975). Thresholds of response to electric shock in previously undernourished rats. *Brit. J. Nutr.* **34**, 511–516.

16. Lynch, A. (1976). Passive avoidance behavior and response thresholds in adult male rats after early postnatal undernutrition. *Physiol. Behav.* **16**, 27–32.

17. Bronfenbrenner, U. (1968). Early deprivation in mammals: a cross-species analysis. *In* "Early Experience and Behavior" (G. Newton and S. Levine, eds) pp. 627–764. Thomas, Springfield, IL.

18. Smart, J. L. and Dobbing J. (1977). Increased thirst and hunger in adult rats undernourished as infants: an alternative explanation. *Brit. J. Nutr.* **37**, 421–430.

19. Smart, J. L. (1981). Undernutrition and aggression. *In* "Multidisciplinary Approaches to Aggression Research" (P. F. Brain and D. Benton, eds). pp. 179–191. Elsevier/North Holland, Amsterdam.

20. Barnett, S. A., Smart, J. L. and Widdowson, E. M. (1971). Early nutrition and the activity and feeding of rats in an artificial environment. *Devl Psychobiol.* **4**, 1–15.

21. Slob, A. K., Snow, C. E. and De Natris-Mathot. E. (1973). Absence of behavioral deficits following neonatal undernutrition in the rat. *Devl Psychobiol.* **6**, 177–186.

22. Dobbing, J. and Smart, J. L. (1974). Vulnerability of developing brain and behaviour. *Brit. Med. Bull.* **30**, 164–168.
23. Donaldson, H. H. (1924). "The Rat. Data and Reference Tables", 2nd edn, Memoirs of the Wistar Institute of Anatomy and Biology, No. 6. Wistar Institute, Philadelphia.
24. Stein, Z., Susser, M., Saenger, G. and Marolla, F. (1975). "Famine and Human Development. The Dutch Hunger Winter of 1944–1945." Oxford University Press, New York.
25. Ross, M. H. (1976). Nutrition and longevity in experimental animals. *In* "Nutrition and Aging" (M. Winick, ed.) pp. 43–57. Wiley, New York.
26. Harper, A. E. (1982). Nutrition, aging and longevity. *Amer. J. Clin. Nutr.* **36** (No. 4 Suppl.) 737–749.
27. Masoro, E. J. (1985). Nutrition and aging—a current assessment. *J. Nutr.* **115**, 842–848.
28. Widdowson, E. M. and Kennedy, G. C. (1962). Rate of growth, mature weight and life span. *Proc. Roy. Soc. B.* **156**, 96–108.
29. Smart, J. L. Animal models of early malnutrition: advantages and limitations. *In* "Malnutrition and Behavior: Critical Assessment of Key Issues" (J. Brožek and B. Schürch, eds) pp. 444–459. Nestlé Foundation, Lausanne, Switzerland.
30. Cowley, J. J. and Griesel, R. D. (1959). Some effects of a low protein diet on a first filial generation of white rats. *J. Genet. Psychol.* **95**, 187–201.
31. Platt, B. S. and Stewart, R. J. C. (1968). Effect of protein–calorie deficiency on dogs. I. Reproduction, growth, and behaviour. *Devl Med. Child Neurol.* **10**, 3–24.
32. Stewart, R. J. C., Preece, R. F. and Sheppard, H. G. (1975). Twelve generations of marginal protein deficiency. *Brit. J. Nutr.* **33**, 233–253.
33. Stewart, R. J. C., Sheppard, H., Preece, R. and Waterlow, J. C. (1980). The effect of rehabilitation at different stages of development of rats marginally malnourished for ten to twelve generations. *Brit. J. Nutr.* **43**, 403–412.
34. Galler, J. R. (1981). Visual discrimination in rats: the effects of rehabilitation following intergenerational malnutrition. *Devl Psychobiol.* **14**, 229–236.
35. Cowley, J. J. and Griesel, R. D. (1966). The effect on growth and behaviour of rehabilitating first and second generation low protein rats. *Anim. Behav.* **14**, 506–517.
36. Galler, J. R. and Propert, K. J. (1981). Maternal behavior following rehabilitation of rats with intergenerational malnutrition. 1. Persistent changes in lactation-related behaviors. *J. Nutr.* **111**, 1330–1336.
37. Lloyd-Still, J. D., Hurwitz, I., Wolff, P. H. and Shwachman, H. (1974). Intellectual development after severe malnutrition in infancy. *Pediatrics* **54**, 306–311.
38. Ellis, C. E. and Hill, D. E. (1975). Growth, intelligence and school performance in children with cystic fibrosis who have had an episode of malnutrition during infancy. *J. Pediat.* **87**, 565–567.
39. Klein, P. S., Forbes, G. B. and Nader, P. R. (1975). Effects of starvation in infancy (pyloric stenosis) on subsequent learning abilities. *J. Pediat.* **87**, 8–15.
40. Dobbing, J. (1981). The later development of the brain and its vulnerability. *In* "Scientific Foundations of Paediatrics," 2nd edn. (J. A. Davis and J. Dobbing, eds) pp. 744–759. Heinemann, London.
41. Hertzig, M. E., Birch, H. G., Richardson, S. A. and Tizard, J. (1972). Intellectual levels of school children severely malnourished during the first two years of life. *Pediatrics* **49**, 814–824.

42. Galler, J. R., Ramsey, F., Solimano, G., Lowell, W. E. and Mason, E. (1983). The influence of early malnutrition on subsequent behavioral development. I. Degree of impairment of intellectual performance. *J. Amer. Acad. Child Psychiat.* **22**, 8–15.

43. Freeman, H. E., Klein, R. E., Townsend, J. W. and Lechtig, A. (1980). Nutrition and cognitive development among rural Guatemalan children. *Amer. J. Publ. Hlth* **70**, 1277–1285.

44. Richardson, S. A. (1976). The relation of severe malnutrition in infancy to the intelligence of school children with differing life histories. *Pediat. Res.* **10**, 57–61.

45. Richardson, S. A., Koller, H., Katz, M. and Albert, K. (1978). The contributions of differing degrees of acute and chronic malnutriton to the intellectual development of Jamaican boys. *Early Human Dev.* **2**, 163–170.

46. Galler, J. R., Ramsey, F. and Solimano, G. (1984). The influence of early malnutrition on subsequent behavioral development. III. Learning disabilities as a sequel to malnutrition. *Pediat. Res.* **18**, 309–313.

47. Freud, S. (1933). "New Introductory Lectures on Psychoanalysis." Norton, New York.

48. Hunt, J. M. (1941). The effects of infant feeding-frustration upon adult hoarding in the albino rat. *J. Abnorm. Soc. Psychol.* **36**, 338–360.

49. Hebb, D. O. (1949). "The Organization of Behavior." Wiley, New York.

50. Bernstein, L. (1952). A note on Christie's "Experimental naiveté and experiential naiveté". *Psychol. Bull.* **49**, 38–40.

51. Weininger, O. (1953). Mortality of albino rats under stress as a function of early handling. *Canad. J. Psychol.* **7**, 111–114.

52. Newton, G. and Levine, S. (eds) (1968). "Early Experience and Behavior." Thomas, Springfield, IL.

53. Schaefer, T. (1968). Some methodological implications of the research on "early handling" in the rat. *In* "Early Experience and Behavior" (G. Newton and S. Levine, eds) pp. 102–141. Thomas, Springfield, IL.

54. Russell, P. A. (1971). "Infantile stimulation" in rodents: a consideration of possible mechanisms. *Psychol. Bull.* **75**, 192–202.

55. Ressler, R. H. (1963). Genotype-correlated parental influences in two strains of mice. *J. Comp. Physiol. Psychol.* **56**, 882–886.

56. Young, R. D. (1965). Influence of neonatal treatment on maternal behavior: a confounding variable. *Psychonom. Sci.* **3**, 295–296.

57. Barnett, S. A. and Burn, J. (1967). Early stimulation and maternal behaviour. *Nature, Lond.* **213**, 150–152.

58. Fraňková, S. (1968). Nutritional and psychological factors in the development of spontaneous behavior in the rat. *In* "Malnutrition, Learning and Behavior" (N. S. Scrimshaw and J. E. Gordon, eds) pp. 312–322. MIT Press, Cambridge, MA.

59. Smart, J. L., Katz, H. B. and Stephens, D. N. (1981). Growth and development of artificially reared well-fed and underfed rats. *Proc. Nutr. Soc.* **40**, 64A.

60. Plaut, S. M. (1970). Studies of undernutrition in the young rat: methodological considerations. *Devl Psychobiol.* **3**, 157–167.

61. Fraňková, S. (1971). Relationship between nutrition during lactation and maternal behaviour of rats. *Activ. Nerv. Sup., Praha.* **13**, 1–8.

62. Smart, J. L. and Preece, J. (1973). Maternal behaviour of undernourished mother rats. *Anim. Behav.* **21**, 613–619.

63. Massaro, T. F., Levitsky, D. A. and Barnes, R. H. (1974). Protein malnutrition in the rat: its effects on maternal behavior and pup development. *Devl Psychobiol* **7**, 551–561.

64. Crnic, L. S. (1976). Maternal behavior in the undernourished rat (*Rattus norvegicus*). *Physiol. Behav.* **16**, 677–680.
65. Misanin, J. R., Hommel, M. J. and Krieger, W. G. (1979). Effect of pup undernutrition on the retrieval behavior of the rat dam. *Behav. Neural Biol.* **27**, 115–119.
66. Smart, J. L. (1980). Attempts at equivalent maternal care for well-fed and underfed offspring: are the problems appreciated? *Devl Psychobiol.* **13**, 431–433.
67. Crnic, L. S. (1980). Models of infantile malnutrition in rats: effects on maternal behavior. *Devl Psychobiol.* **13**, 615–628.
68. Smart, J. L., Stephens, D. N. and Katz, H. B. (1983). Growth and development of rats artificially reared on a high or a low plane of nutrition. *Brit. J. Nutr.* **49**, 497–506.
69. Turkewitz, G. (1984). Animal models or the comparative approach: a useful distinction in studying malnutrition and behavior. *In* "Malnutrition and Behavior: Critical Assessment of Key Issues" (J. Brožek and B. Schürch, eds) pp. 469–473. Nestlé Foundation, Lausanne, Switzerland.
70. Villescas, R., Zamenhof, S. and Guthrie, D. (1979). The effects of early stress and undernutrition on the behavior of young adult rats and the correlations between behavioral and brain parameters. *Physiol. Behav.* **23**, 945–954.
71. Crnic, L. S. (1983). Effects of nutrition and environment on brain biochemistry and behavior. *Devl Psychobiol.* **16**, 129–145.
72. Swanson, H. H., McConnell, F., Uylings, H. B. M., Van Oyen, H. G. and Van de Poll, N. E. (1983). Interaction between pre-weaning undernutrition and post-weaning environmental enrichment on somatic development and behaviour in male and female rats. *Behav. Processes* **8**, 1–20.
73. Smart, J. L. (1986). Undernutrition, learning and memory: review of experimental studies. *In* "Proceedings of the XIIIth International Congress of Nutrition" (T. G. Taylor and N. K. Jenkins, eds) pp. 74–78. Libbey, London.
74. Richardson, S. A., Birch, H. G. and Ragbeer, C. (1975). The behaviour of children at home who were severely malnourished in the first 2 years of life. *J. Biosoc. Sci.* **7**, 255–267.
75. Seligman, M. E. P. (1975). "Helplessness." W. H. Freeman & Co., San Francisco, CA.
76. Winick, M. (1970). Cellular growth in intrauterine malnutrition. *Pediat. Clin. N. Amer.* **17**, 69–78.

Commentary

Linda S. Crnic: As usual, I find little to disagree with in Smart's analysis of the field of non-human animal research on the effects of malnutrition. I do feel that he is a bit too modest about the accomplishments of his own and others' research. In stating that no major breakthroughs have occurred in animal research, he neglects an important "discovery" which has had long-lasting impact the treatment of human malnutrition. I refer to the realization of the importance of environmental factors which invariably accompany malnutrition. This is an important point which is emphasized by each of the other chapters in the volume. This point is most strikingly presented in Sinisterra's paper (this volume). Having tried, with success, various educational interventions with malnourished children, Sinisterra's group has turned their attention to interventions designed to have a much more comprehensive impact upon the total environment of the child. The importance of the realization that food alone is not the remedy to malnutrition cannot be overemphasized.

The discovery of the importance of environmental factors illustrates the type of interaction between human and animal researchers that Smart advocates in the end of his paper. As he notes, there has been interaction between animal and human research on this topic. It is important to see that this type of interaction must be extended to all levels of research. It is artificial and non-productive to view different approaches to any problem in science as separate or competitive. I prefer to conceptualize all research as existing on a continuum: at one extreme lies the most basic research into the subatomic structure of matter and at the other extreme, the study of the sociology of whole societies. None of the types of research along the continuum can exist independently, and each type of research is necessary in solving important scientific problems (1). Interaction must occur between many levels of research. The study of malnutrition illustrates this nicely. Research with humans is necessary to define the problem in humans and to develop hypotheses. It is then necessary to call upon extensive knowledge of animal behaviour and development in order to choose an appropriate model. Techniques from other levels of analysis, such as the neuroscience techniques described by Bedi in this volume, must then be brought into play to produce data. These data then can result in hypotheses which can be tested in humans. The work of Sinisterra reaches toward the other end of the continuum: he describes how study of the individual has led to intervention involving the whole family, and makes it obvious that the eventual solutions to the problems of malnutrition rest ultimately at the level of national and global politics. He states that this is beyond the purview of science, but I suspect that the economists and sociologists would disagree with this assessment. Indeed, perhaps significant progress can be made in eliminating childhood malnutrition only when we acknowledge the need for the expertise of these social scientists.

Another aspect of the environment/nutrition issue raised by Smart is the interaction between the two factors. This is one of the few areas of agreement in the research on the effects of malnutrition. Although the experiments use a variety of methods for producing malnutrition and measure a variety of outcomes, the overwhelming consensus is that environmental enrichment has beneficial effects upon behaviour and brain measures (refs 2-22 support this conclusion, 23 and 24 do not). These studies also conclude that environmental enrichment does not completely eliminate the effects of malnutrition, in part because the two treatments affect different variables. A careful analysis of the actual data from the many animal experiments that address this topic produces interesting conclusions about the interaction between nutrition and environment. The nature of this interaction is properly addressed only in those studies in which normal (if any laboratory environment can be said to be normal), in addition to impoverished and enriched environments are studied. The reason for this is illustrated in Fig. 1. As the figure shows, it is possible that the effects of impoverishment interact differently with nutrition than do the effects of enrichment. Indeed, the data indicates that impoverishment can have a larger effect upon malnourished animals than well nourished animals (16), while the opposite seems to be true of enrichment: malnourished animals are less (6,11) or equally (2–5,7,9,10,12–15,18) affected as well

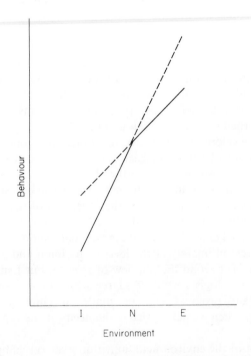

Fig. 1. Hypothetical interaction between nutrition and environment. The two lines represent two nutritional conditions, for example well nourished and malnourished. I, impoverished; N, normal; E, enriched. This figure illustrates the need for three environmental conditions to determine interaction effects. Using only the I and E conditions would lead to the false conclusion that there is no interaction between nutrition and environment.

nourished animals by environmental enrichment. Thus, if one studies only the two extremes, one risks missing an interaction effect between the two variables.

My only objection to Smart's paper is that, perhaps for lack of space to explain the complicated issues, he has painted too optimistic a picture of the advantages of animal research. While many things can be controlled in animal research, it is still important to realize that the effects of malnutrition are always confounded with environmental changes, and thus one can never separate environmental from nutritional effects. This is because maternal behaviour is determined in part by the physical and behavioural characteristics of the offspring (e.g. 25). To the extent that malnutrition alters those characteristics by making the offspring less mature and less vigorous, maternal behaviour, an important component of the environment, is altered (26).

1. Crnic, L. S., Reite, M. L. and Shucard, D. W. (1982). Animal models of human behavior: Their application to the study of attachment. *In* "Attachment and Affiliative Systems: Neurobiological and Psychobiological Aspects" (R. N. Emde and R. Harmon, eds) pp. 31–42. Plenum Press, New York.
2. Bhide, P. G. and Bedi, K. S. (1982). The effects of environmental diversity on well-fed and previously undernourished rats. I. Body and brain measurements. *J. Comp. Neurol.* **207**, 403–409.
3. Bhide, P. G. and Bedi, K. S. (1984). The effects of a lengthy period of environmental diversity on well-fed and previously undernourished rats. I. Neurons and glial cells. *J. Comp. Neurol.* **227**, 296–304.
4. Bhide, P. G. and Bedi, K. S. (1984). The effects of environmental diversity on well fed and previously undernourished rats: neuronal and glial cell measurements in the visual cortex (area 17). *J. Anat.* **138**, 447–461.
5. Celedon, J. M., Santander, M. and Colombo, M. (1979). Long-term effects of early undernutrition and environmental stimulation on learning performance of adult rats. *J. Nutr.* **109**, 1880–1886.
6. Cines, B. M. and Winick, M. (1979). Behavioral and physiological effects of early handling and early malnutrition in rats. *Devl Psychobiol.* **12**, 381–389.
7. Davies, C. A. and Katz, H. B. (1973). The comparative effects of early-life undernutrition and subsequent differential environmental on the dendritic branching of pyramidal cells in rat visual cortex. *J. Comp. Neurol.* **218**, 345–350.
8. Eckert, C. D., Levitsky, D. A. and Barnes, R. H. (1975). Postnatal stimulation: The effects on cholinergic enzyme activity in undernourished rats. *Proc. Soc. Exp. Biol. Med.* **149**, 860–863.
9. Elias, M. F. and Samonds, K. W. (1972). Interactive effects of nutritional and rearing deprivation on activity and exploratory behavior in infant monkeys. *Fed. Proc.* **32**, 909.
10. Fraňková, (1968). Nutritional and psychological factors in the development of spontaneous behavior in the rat. *In* "Malnutrition, Learning and Behavior" (N. S. Scrimshaw and J. E. Gordon, eds). MIT Press, Cambridge, MA.
11. Fraňková, S. (1972). Influence of nutrition and early experience on behaviour of rats. *Biblio. Nutritio et Dieta.* **17**, 96–110.
12. Katz, H. B. and Davies, C. A. (1982). The effects of early-life undernutrition and subsequent environmental on morphological parameters of the rat brain. *Behav. Brain Res.* **5**, 53–64.

13. Katz, H. B. and Davies, C. A. (1983). The separate and combined effects of early undernutrition and environmental complexity at different ages on cerebral measures in rats. *Devl Psychobiol.* **16**, 47–58.
14. Katz, H. B., Davies, C. A. and Dobbing, J. (1980). The effect of environmental stimulation on brain weight in previously undernourished rats. *Behav. Brain Res.* **1**, 445–449.
15. Katz, H. B., Davies, C. A. and Dobbing, J. (1982). Effects of undernutrition at different ages early in life and later environmental complexity on parameters of cerebrum and hippocampus in rats. *J. Nutr* **112**, 1362–1368.
16. Levitsky, D. A. and Barnes, R. H. (1972). Nutritional and environmental interactions in the behavioral development of the rat: long-term effects. *Science* **176**, 68–71.
17. Morgan, B. L. G. and Winick, M. (1980). Effects of environmental stimulation on brain N-acetylneuraminic acid content and behavior. *J. Nutr.* **110**, 415–432.
18. Sara, V. R., King, T. L. and Lazarus, L. (1976). The influence of early nutrition and environmental rearing on brain growth and behavior. *Experientia* **32**, 1538–1540.
19. Slob, A. K., Snow, C. E. and deNatris-Mathot, E. (1973). Absense of behavioral deficits following neonatal undernutrition in the rat. *Devl Psychobiol.* **6**, 177–186.
20. Tanabe, G. (1972). Remediating maze deficiencies by the use of environmental enrichment. *Devl Psychol.* **7**, 244.
21. Vore, D. A. and Ottinger, D. R. (1970). Maternal food restriction: Effects of offspring development, learning, and a program of therapy. *Devl Psychobiol.* **3**, 337–342.
22. Wells, A. M., Geist, C. R. and Zimmerman, R. R. (1972). Influence of environmental and nutritional factors on problem solving in the rat. *Percept. Motor Skills* **3**, 235–244.
23. Leathwood, P. D., Bush, M. S. and Mauron, J. (1975). The effects of Chlordiazepoxide on avoidance performance of mice subjected to undernutrition or handling stress in early life. *Psychopharm.* **41**, 105–110.
24. Cines, B. M. (1976). Effects of early handling and early malnutrition on developmental changes in the open field behavior of rats. *Diss. Abstr.* **37**, 1402.
25. Rosenblatt, J. S. (1965). The basis of synchrony in the behavioral interaction between the mother and offspring in the laboratory rats. *In* "Determinants of Infant Behavior III" (B. M. Foss, ed.) pp. 3–41. Methuen, London.
26. Smart, J. L. (1980). Comment: attempts at equivalent maternal care for well-fed and underfed offspring: are the problems appreciated? *Devl Psychobiol.* **13**, 431–434.

D. E. Barrett: Smart's paper gives a concise analysis of the ways in which animal research studies contribute to our understanding of the possible effects of early malnutrition. I think he is precisely correct in his concluding statement that what the field researcher on human malnutrition can learn from the animal research is that "this possible aspect of behaviour" or "this possible mechanism" (whereby early malnutrition may affect behaviour) may be worthy of study in the field.

I drew directly from the animal research in generating hypotheses about the long-term effects of chronic undernutrition, and, specifically, in considering what aspects of behaviour and what mediating processes would be implicated (1,2). My reliance on animal studies was criticized by Super (3) who stated that my assumption seemed to be—to paraphrase—"This occurs for animals so why not for humans?"

Of course it would be foolish to assume that one can generalize a documented causal influence (for example, of a nutritional insult on a behaviour impairment) across species without some supporting evidence. But it not only makes sense; it is our responsibility to use the comparative research to generate theoretical models and test them.

Our research findings linking a history of chronic energy deficit to low social involvement, distractability, lack of persistence on difficult problems, and reduced initiative and exploration in children were made possible by a clear theoretical base generated from the animal research.

I disagree with Smart's statement that there have been no "breakthroughs" in the field of research on the effects of malnutrition on animal behaviour. Perhaps I am naive, but as a post-doctoral fellow ten years ago, first considering the possibility of the study of the effects of malnutrition on social development, I found that Levitsky and Barnes' concept of "functional isolation" (4) was extremely important in helping to understand the behavioural implications of malnutrition. I would say now that the concept of "functional isolation" is an *organizing construct* of the highest order—a theoretically compelling as well as clinically appealing construct from which we have been able to generate testable hypotheses and theories. Not only has this idea been useful in helping us to understand the sequellae of early undernutrition, it has been helpful in considering clinical management of failure-to-thrive and also in looking for behavioural indicators of early organic insult. Deborah Frank (5) discusses the relationship of the research on protein–energy malnutrition to the understanding of non-organic failure-to-thrive.

Finally, I would call attention to the following passage in Smart's paper, one which contains, I believe, a flaw in interpretation but is important because of the conclusion ultimately drawn:

> . . . Social behavior can be qualitatively different between species . . . Hence, it is probably not surprising that there is no correspondence between the heightened social reactivity in undernourished rats . . . and the unsociable, withdrawn behavior of formerly malnourished Jamaican children . . . What is noteworthy, however, is that social behavior was affected, somehow, in both man and rat. (p. 66)

It is indeed noteworthy, and, on theoretical and empirical grounds would have been predicted. Smart sees it as an inconsistency that heightened reactivity has been found in rats and lessened reactivity in children. In fact, the findings are linked by the notion of inappropriate emotional response to moderate stress or challenge (i.e. such that there is an interference with normal adaptive response). The finding that social behaviour is affected in both species should not be viewed as problematic. (Smart's qualifier "somehow" suggests that the finding is important but puzzling.)

The research on malnutrition and emotional response is consistent in showing, across species, that malnourished animals manifest interfering emotional responses (be they in terms of under- or over-reactivity) to stimulus situations which would be better served by more well-modulated responses. Thus, both the inhibition of early malnourished animals in exploratory situations (6,7) and the overly active behaviours of malnourished animals in certain learning situations (8) indicate what Wiener and colleagues describe as failures in "coping" (9).

I have argued that our failure to conceptualize our constructs (e.g. emotionality) carefully has led to situations where investigators treat data which may in fact be highly consistent as though they were contradictory.

Again, that social behaviour is affected is not only noteworthy, it is theoretically predicted (see 1,2 and my paper in this volume).

1. Barrett, D. E., Radke-Yarrow, M. and Klein, R. E. (1982). Chronic malnutrition and child behavior: Effects of early caloric supplementation on social and emotional functioning at school age. *Devl Psychol.* **18**, 541–556.
2. Barrett, D. E. and Radke-Yarrow, M. (1985). Effects of nutritional supplementation on children's responses to novel, frustrating and competitive situations. *Amer. J. Clin. Nutr.* **42**, 102–120.
3. Super, C. M. (1984). Models of assessment and development. *In* "Malnutrition and Behavior: A Critical Assessment of Key Issues" (J. Brožek and B. Schürch, eds) pp. 327–336. Foundation, Lausanne, Switzerland.
4. Levitsky, D. A. and Barnes, R. H. (1972). Nutritional and environmental interactions in the behavioral development of the rat: long-term effects. *Science* **176**, 68–71.
5. Frank, D. A. (1984). Malnutrition and child behavior: a view from the bedside. *In* "Malnutrition and Behavior: A Critical Assessment of Key Issues" (J. Brožek and B. Schürch, eds) pp. 307–326. Nestlé Foundation, Lausanne, Switzerland.
6. Barnes, R. H., Levitsky, D. A., Pond, W. G. and Moore, U. (1975). Effects of postnatal dietary deprivation and energy restriction on exploratory behavior in young pigs. *Devl Psychobiol.* **9**, 425–435.
7. Zimmerman, R. R., Strobel, D. A. and McGuire, D. (1979). Neophobic reactions in protein malnourished infant monkeys. *Proc. 78th Ann. Conv. APA* **6**, 197.
8. Fraňková, S. and Barnes, R. H. (1968). Effect of malnutrition in early life on avoidance conditioning and behavior of adult rats. *J. Nutr.* **96**, 485–493.
9. Wiener, S. G., Robinson, L. and Levine, S. (1983). Influence of perinatal malnutrition on adult physiological and behavioral reactivity in rats. *Physiol. Behav.* **30**, 41–50.

Author's reply: Barrett disagrees with my assessment that there have been "no breakthroughs" in the field of early malnutrition and behaviour. He cites Levitsky and Barnes's functional isolation hypothesis as a breakthrough and writes of it as "theoretically compelling" and an "organizing construct of the highest order". (For a brief description of the hypothesis see Levitsky and Strupp's commentary on Galler's paper (this volume). Levitsky and Strupp's "software hypothesis" is the same as the "functional isolation hypothesis", as I understand it.) The disagreement is probably in the degree to which we have been seduced by the idea. I state that the hypothesis has been influential and has stimulated a considerable amount of experimentation. To me the idea was, and still is, an interesting hypothesis to be tested. To Barrett, it seems to be a concept which has restructured his thinking about the world of early malnutrition. I shall reserve the restructuring of my ideas until the hypothesis is fully tested. It may be correct, incorrect or, most likely, partly correct. Some attempts to test the hypothesis are described and discussed by Rogers *et al.* (1).

1. Rogers, P. J., Smart, J. L. and Tonkiss, J. (1986). Incidental learning is impaired during early-life undernutrition. *Devl. Psychobiol.* **19**, 113–124.

I. Hurwitz: H. G. Taylor of the University of Pittsburg Medical School wrote in 1984 that "the gap between understanding human behavior and its underpinnings in neurophysiology has yet to be bridged" (1). It has long been suggested that a vital strategy for achieving success in constructing this metaphorical bridge is through the use of animal models. A review of two widely used textbooks in university courses in physiological psychology, Carlson's *Physiology of Behavior* and Grover and Schlesinger's *Biological Psychology* demonstrates clearly the substantial reliance on the results of animal experiments in the entire spectrum of brain functions which have been studied. Indeed, it would be an exercise in redundancy to cite the list of awards which neuroscientists have garnered for their work with animal populations, such that there is literally no margin of argument or dispute to the relevancy and importance of this research technique to advancing our understanding of a variety of phenomena. It is an approach which certainly merits the term indispensable as a component of the research armamentarium. It has enabled investigators to explore the suspected, adverse effect of a variety of noxious agents and conditions involving lead ingestion, atmospheric carbon monoxide, protracted isolation, or selective exclusion of various sensory and perceptual experience, etc. Significant applications in public health and therapeutic activities and programmes have originated in the work carried out in animal laboratories, efforts which have had far-reaching implications for society at large. Yet despite the many advantages and opportunities which animal studies present, there are clearly large areas of ambiguity and doubt as to their full utility in studies of undernutrition effects, even when one is seeking analogues or parallels with human behaviour at the social or intellectual level. Animal studies are nevertheless best used to understand mechanisms of function in a system, rather than as the basis for extrapolated consequences of functions observed in broader behavioural terms (2). Thus animal studies may increase our knowledge of morphological changes (Bedi, this volume) biochemical changes (3) and electrophysiological changes (4). When similar psychological functions can be identified such as memory or social behaviour, certain analogies between humans and animals can be defined in controlled experimental conditions and indeed, a voluminous literature exists on this topic, not only with respect to undernutrition or malnutrition as independent variables, but with a wide variety of antecedent conditions as well.

In a recent discussion of an earlier article dealing with the advantages and shortcomings of animal models by Smart (5), Crnic states, "Dr Smart's very thorough review . . . leaves little else to be said on the topic." I would certainly agree with this assessment and apply it in the context of the present article. It encompasses virtually all the important issues both in favour and opposed to this technique. However, I was especially interested in Smart's specific definition of what in his view, would in fact constitute a genuine animal model. He states "a more precise usage is to restrict the term to experiments in which an attempt has been made to mimic some human condition or situation." In this connection he cites transgenerational undernutrition in man as the repeatable experimental condition which can be created in the laboratory rat, and from which findings relevant to influences on problem solving, learning, and maternal behaviour "have important implications for social and economic planning". I would interpret this to mean that the conclusions we would draw from the effects of transgenerational under-nutrition and malnutrition are that rehabilitation, to be effective, through supplementation, for example, must go beyond its availability to a single generation. This seems hardly a surprising conclusion to be derived from so complex a design.

I would suggest that a true animal model of conditions which reflect the social circumstances surrounding human undernutrition would be one in which overcrowding, excessive noise, inconsistent parental care, exposure to infection, unclean cages, and insufficient attention to general health needs would be the baseline of experimental circumstances into which varying degrees of undernutrition would be introduced, and then measures would be taken of effects after whatever manipulations of timing, duration, protein and/or energy deficits were introduced. It becomes increasingly discouraging and even tiresome to read the repetitive emphasis in animal study reports on the seemingly inevitable lack of precision in measurement, the neglect of methodological rules and appropriate statistical measures, the differences in species responses in which one species (the rat) shows too much of a response that another species (man) shows too little of, and then to speculate as to the basis for this disparity when the reason becomes patently clear in the obvious fact that they are inherently different organisms, studied under fundamentally different conditions, despite the fact that the samples of both groups have been exposed to the same experience — namely, undernutrition. Even with animal models as a means of accomplishing a whole host of studies which could not be carried out with humans, it was still impossible to conclude that deficits in "brain growth" were alone responsible for the deficits in behaviour resulting from, or at least following, periods of malnutrition and undernutrition. The search for neural mechanism while essential, becomes more and more frustrated by massive methodological problems leading Smart to conclude: "The question remains whether there are lasting effects of early undernutrition on behaviour, which are mediated *directly* (his italics) through restriction of brain growth. It is debatable whether or not this can be answered unequivocally . . ."

In the final analysis, it is difficult to go beyond the so-called "cautions" which Smart presents without a sense of unease about the value of animal models in this field. It seems a somewhat minimal contribution to our fund of knowledge to state that increased social responsiveness in the nutritionally rehabilitated rat on the one hand, and withdrawal and poor sociability in the once malnourished Jamaican children studied on the other, mean that there is "some kind of effect for the likes of social behaviour" following upon early exposure to undernutrition.

Crnic's (6) statement that animal studies were not carried out to answer the questions of quantity or extent of behavioural effects of malnutrition, but rather to deal with questions about mechanisms, seems to make the most sense. That the eventual value of such research one expects will be to indicate where remedies and rehabilitative efforts are to be most productively directed appears to be a most reasonable conclusion.

1. Taylor, H. G. (1984). Neuropsychological approaches to children: towards a developmental neuropsychology. *J. Clin. Neuropsychol.* **6**, 39–56.
2. Crnic, L. S. (1984). Animal models of early malnutrition: A comment on bias, dependability and human importance. *In* "Malnutrition and Behavior: A Critical Assessment of Key Issues" (J. Brožek and B. Schürch, eds). Nestlé Foundation, Lausanne, Switzerland.
3. Crnic, L. S. *op. cit.*
4. Griesel, R. D. (ed.) (1980). "Malnutrition in Southern Africa." University of South Africa, Pretoria.
5. Smart, J. L. (1984). Animal models of early malnutrition: advantages and limitations. *In* "Malnutrition and Behavior: A Critical Assessment of Key Issues" (J. Brožek and B. Schürch, eds). Nestlé Foundation, Lausanne, Switzerland.
6. Crnic, L. S. *op. cit.*

Author's reply: It is hard to disagree with any specific aspect of Hurwitz's commentary, only with its general tone. He seems to have viewed the paper through a rather sombre, pessimistic filter, which emphasizes the limitations of the animal work while detracting from its advantages and potential value.

With respect to the research on multigenerational malnutrition in rats, I should have said that it was a partial model of the human situation or, as I did state in my Conclusions (p. 68), a ". . . model of one facet of the human situation". Hurwitz is right to point out that, in order to mimic the human condition, the model would have to include such environmental conditions as overcrowding, noise and pollution in addition to malnutrition. How useful this would be would depend on the question under investigation. One would learn nothing about the effects of transgenerational malnutrition from such a model alone. Whether or not Hurwitz finds the results of multigenerational malnutrition studies surprising, seems to me neither here nor there. Surely we are not going to put a greater value on surprising findings than on unsurprising ones? What matters is how appropriate the questions are, and to what extent the experiments answer them.

Sally Grantham McGregor: Smart points out that whereas only 22% of the variance in the composite cognitive score was explained in the Guatemalan study (1), 45% of the variance in IQ scores was explained in the Jamaican study (2). He attributes the difference to "finer grained analysis" in the Jamaican study. It is probable that differences in the age and type of population may be responsible. In Guatemala (1) the population was a homogeneous cohort of undernourished village children, whereas in the Jamaican study (2) there were two distinct groups of children different in nutritional status and social background.

Smart's hypothesis that relatively minor factors may have important effects on mental development when interacting with other factors is interesting, and one we have thought about for some time. It could be, for instance, that iron deficiency anaemia or exposure to low lead levels, are more detrimental in malnourished children than in normal children.

If we wish to extrapolate to the human, studies which copy the human condition as closely as possible should be the most useful. However, what puzzles me is that there seems little serious attempt to do this. For instance malnourished children generally have diets which are primarily calorie deficient, and protein deficient diets are uncommon. In addition malnourished children are usually exposed to overcrowded and noisy environments, not isolated ones, and they rarely return to good diets following an acute episode but spend the rest of their childhood on marginal diets. I realize that I am ignorant in the field of animal reseach and perhaps there are good reasons why models like these are not usually attempted.

1. Freeman, H. E., Klein, R. E., Townsend, J. W. and L. Lechtig, A. (1980). Nutrition and cognitive development among rural Guatemalan children. *Amer. J. Publ. Hlth.* **70**, 1277–1285.
2. Richardson, S. A. (1976). The relation of severe malnutrition in infancy to the intelligence of school children with differing life histories. *Pediat. Res.* **10**, 57–61.

J. Dobbing: I think that to ask for animal studies to "mimic the human condition as closely as possible" is to ask for the impossible, and at the same time misses one of the main potential strengths of the animal experimental method. The heterogeneity of human children, with their widely differing nutritional and experiential history, itself leads to the need for a more controlled analysis of the various factors; and it is this which animals can help to provide. There are very few animal experimental designs in any field which can exactly copy human circumstances. I believe it to be a common feature of a blinkered attitude that is part of the clinician's training and experience, to decry the proper use of animals which can, on occasions, illuminate the human problem more effectively than direct study; simply because of the sheer complexity and heterogeneity of people. The question whether nutrition has any role in future human achievement will never be answered by human studies. Animal experiment has the potential to come much closer because of its greater analytical power, although it, too, will never provide the ultimate answer to a question like this, perhaps because it is too simplistically posed.

D. A. Levitsky and Barbara J. Strupp: In his paper, Smart argues that one value of animal research is that it allows the study of the effects of malnutrition on brain where such research is difficult, if not impossible, to do in humans. Although we totally agree with Smart, we believe that his description underestimates the importance of studying animals. Not only can the effects of malnutrition on brain structures (as described so well by Bedi) and brain chemistry be more rigorously examined in animals than in humans, but more precise correlations can be calculated between the changes in brain with the alteration in behaviour.

Unlike human research, the behaviour of experimental animals can be continually assessed until sacrifice. Also, large numbers of subjects can be used for each experiment. Such conditions allow behaviour to be intensely studied in one group of animals while another, identically treated group, can be used for brain analysis. Systematically correlating alterations in specific brain structure and chemistry to changes in behaviour can provide direction towards those particular brain processes that might be responsible for the changes in the behaviour or cognition, as well as provide information as to what brain changes may *not* be involved in producing abnormal behaviour. We must not forget that the brain contains a large amount of redundancy, and the mere decrease of tissue or metabolites does not necessarily constitute dysfunction. By understanding what processes are and are not correlated with behavioural change we will improve our understanding of the brain structures and chemical processes responsible for determining brain function to a far greater degree than can be obtained by only studying human brain injury.

The practice of raising laboratory animals in a "simple, unvarying and unchallenging" environment is widespread. The purpose of using an "impoverished" environment is to minimize the influence of many uncontrolled variables in a study. The consequence, however, is that this environment is not only a poor homology of the human condition, but is extremely foreign to the "natural" development of the animal, even a rat. Even more importantly, raising animals in such environments may actually produce erroneous conclusions concerning the nature of variables on behaviour. For example, normally a young rat, like a young child, lives in an environment in which it is continually exposed to information. A large number of studies have demonstrated that the cognitive capacity of young rodents is greatly enhanced by exposing the young rodent to complex environments, a phenomenon that is easily demonstrated by the increased rate at which they can solve problems.

Because most studies of the effects of malnutrition in animals do not use enriched environments, the performance of the control animals, to which the malnourished, or previously malnourished animals will be compared, will always be less than proficient than animals raised in an enriched environment. Inferring that no difference in cognition exists between malnourished animals and isolated control animals raised in environmentally impoverished environments may be as fallacious as concluding that mentally retarded children have normal intelligence when the control group consists of children raised in closets. Yet, many researchers using animals to study malnutrition, including the authors, have based our assessments of brain function of the malnourished animal on the performance of environmentally isolated controls. We can clearly do better.

There is one further, albeit more abstract, advantage of studying animals. I know of few areas in the neurosciences where more scientists from such diverse backgrounds as psychology, ethology, neuroanatomy, neuro-chemistry, electrophysiology, nutrition, biochemistry, physiology, medicine, and public health come together, without the typical hierarchical condescension of other disciplines, and discuss, plan and work together towards a united goal: to minimize the human suffering from malnutrition.

Such sincere collaboration between disciplines cannot help to advance our understanding of the nature of the influence of nutrition and environment on human growth and development and, consequently, expand our knowledge concerning brain behavioural relationships.

K. S. Bedi: There is not much I can argue with in this very sensibly written paper. Smart has managed to define clearly the purpose and value of experiments on animals in general, and in the field of undernutrition in particular. He points out many of the shortfalls in work on humans who have been unfortunate enough to suffer a period of malnutrition during early life. And yet he maintains a sense of balance as to the limitations of experiments on animals. I hope that this paper is widely read.

The sad thing about this paper is that Smart feels that it is actually necessary to write it in the first place. Is this a reflection of the pressures to which non-clinical scientists feel that they are subjected, both from their clinical colleagues and by activists in the "animal rights" movement? I do not feel that it is the purpose of this workshop to defend animal experimentation against the minority (albeit a vocal minority) of "animal rights" activists. However, there are many clinicians (certainly not all, but nevertheless a significant number) who do decry animal experiments, on the basis that they can have no relevance to humans. This of course is a short-sighted viewpoint. Those who hold it merely display their own limited knowledge and understanding of the scientific process. I do consider it our duty to try to educate such people. I hope Smart's paper will go some way towards this end.

Undernutrition and Child Behaviour: What Behaviours Should We Measure and How Should We Measure Them?

DAVID E. BARRETT

Department of Elementary and Secondary Education, Clemson University, Clemson, SC, USA

What Do We Measure?

A question I am frequently asked by researchers interested in studying the effects of malnutrition or improved nutrition on behaviour is, "What should we use for outcome variables?" The question is a disconcerting one. Outcome variables ("dependent variables") derive from the research question. To find out what outcome variables to measure, the researchers should think about the theoretical rationale for the study, and specifically the hypotheses. If the hypotheses do not suggest the dependent variables, they have not been adequately articulated. If there are no hypotheses, the study should not be carried out for it will not advance our understanding.

The above seems obvious, yet it is astonishing to find how frequently researchers fail to recognize that *only they* know what the dependent variables of their study should be. In fact, I should say that only the researchers themselves know what the dependent variables of the study *are*. The dependent variables are defined by the research question and are stated, at least in general terms, in the hypotheses.

Why has development of dependent variables for research on malnutrition and behaviour been considered a problem? I will address this question in

Early Nutrition and Later Achievement
ISBN: 0-12-218855-1

the following sections. First, however, I would like to define the important terms of this discussion: construct, variable, and measure (measurement). There is one other idea which it is important to understand and that is the (construct) validity of a research design.

Definition of Terms

Construct

A construct is an idea which underlies a measurement operation. It is a theoretical idea which implies individual differences along a continuum or among a set of categories and some way to measure those differences. A construct also implies a network of other constructs (i.e. related ideas) which give it meaning. In psychological research, examples of constructs are "intelligence", "aggression" and "anxiety". In malnutrition research, commonly used constructs are "emotionality", "activity level", and "learning ability".

If, in a research study, we decide to carry out a measurement operation, for example, give an IQ test, we do so because there is a construct underlying our measurement (i.e. intelligence) and we are trying to estimate individual differences on that construct.

What does it mean to say that a construct is given meaning by its relation to other constructs? Let's take, as an example, a construct commonly considered in both the human and animal malnutrition research, and that is "emotionality" (1,2). In most malnutrition research, the investigators have meant by "emotionality" the extent to which the animal or person shows strong emotional responses to tasks or problems which impede successful performance. Suppose an investigator decides to measure emotionality in children by studying their tendency to cry, complain or get angry when trying to solve difficult problems. In conceiving of "emotionality", the investigator must have in mind a "theoretical network" of constructs which give meaning to the construct "emotionality". For example, the investigator might include in this network of constructs ideas such as "attention", "lability of mood", "learning ability", and "achievement", and postulate that attention to tasks and achievement are negatively related to emotionality, lability of mood is positively related, and learning ability is unrelated.

Ideally, the investigator will attempt to build into his research empirical tests of these relationships (3). Failure to identify postulated relationships between the constructs implies one of two things: (a) the theory (set of postulated relationships) is wrong, or (b) the constructs were operationalized inappropriately. Inappropriate operationalization would occur if the measurements were not reliable (i.e. accurate) and/or the measurements were not valid.

Variable

A variable is a characteristic on which people differ. The term "variable" is often used to refer to the construct of interest. For example, an investigator may say that the "dependent variables" in his study were emotionality and activity level and mean, not the operations used to measure those constructs, but the constructs themselves. At other times, researchers use the term variable to refer to measurement procedures. For example, the researcher may say that the dependent variable was 12-month Bayley scores. In saying this, the researcher is referring to the procedures used to study the construct (sensorimotor ability), but not the construct itself. For the present paper, I will use the term variable to refer, at once, to the construct of interest and the procedures used to measure it (whatever those might be).

Measure (Measurement)

When we measure, we assign numbers, values or attributions to things according to rules. When the measurement process is completed, all persons or things to which we wish to assign a value (i.e. subjects) have received one. The number, value or attribute is an estimate of some true amount or quality of the construct of interest. The process of developing measurements from constructs is called the operationalizing of the construct.

As indicated earlier, constructs are theoretically derived. The variables in their operationalized form, that is the measures of the variables, are developed according to both theoretical and psychometric principles. These are discussed further later.

Construct validity of a research design

The most important consideration in evaluating any research design is the construct validity of the design, what Cook and Campbell (4) call "construct validity of putative causes and effects". The construct validity of a design is the extent to which the research design is capable of addressing the theoretical issue which it purports to address. And here is where conceptualization and operationalizing of both independent and dependent variables is important. For if we are not measuring the independent variables (presumed casual or antecedent factors) and the dependent variables (presumed outcome or consequent factors) which are implicit in the research design and the hypotheses, then the study will not address the research question of interest and conclusions will be invalid. For a more detailed discussion of threats to the construct validity of research on the behavioural effects of malnutrition, see Barrett (5).

Why Has Derivation of Appropriate Dependent Variables and Operationalization of Dependent Variables Been Considered a Problem?

In the 1960s and 1970s many studies were published on the effects of malnutrition on children's behaviour. Reviews of this research are in Lloyd-Still (6), Pollitt and Thomson (7) and Barrett and Frank (2), among other works. It has been pointed out, as a criticism of the research, that in most published studies the primary outcome measure is performance on a standardized intelligence test (7,8).

I would agree that up until quite recently, little attention was given to the measurement of other important dimensions of the child's behaviour. I believe that one of the reasons that researchers did not attempt to measure the child's emotional characteristics, ways of interacting with other children, and general social adjustment is that they believed that the most important behaviours are the hardest to measure. (In fact, in his paper written for this workshop*, Sinisterra says, "The social–affective or social–emotional development of young children is particularly hard to measure".) I will discuss this assumption later in the paper. Suffice it to say, for now, that it is an inaccurate assumption but one that many researchers make, and it has led to an emphasis on the use of standardized intelligence tests as outcome measures in research.

The decision to use a standardized intelligence test as the primary dependent variable in studying the behavioural effects of undernutrition or improved nutrition is not necessarily a bad one. In fact, it may be best decision. The important question is: Does the outcome measure I've chosen help me answer the theoretical question I've posed. A second question is: Is this the best measure of the construct that I am interested in?

When is it appropriate to use a standardized intelligence test (IQ test) as an outcome in malnutrition research? When the researcher has hypothesized and *justified on theoretical grounds* a causal relationship between malnutrition and general level of intellectual development (or retardation), then IQ may be used as an outcome variable. That is, if the researchers have (a) hypothesized an effect of the nutritional variable on intelligence and (b) postulated mediating processes by which the nutritional variable could affect intelligence, then the use of a standardized intelligence test as an outcome variable is likely to help them answer the research question of interest. If the researchers have decided to measure IQ *only* because IQ tests are

---

* Sinisterra, L. (1986). Studies of human growth and development: the Cali experience. Paper presented to Early Nutrition and Later Achievement, International Children's Centre, Paris, France, October, 1986.

commonly used, interpretable and known to predict other important outcomes, and not because they have compelling theoretical grounds for predicting an influence of malnutrition on intelligence test performance, then the decision to use IQ as a dependent variable is not a wise one.

In reviewing research on the effects of early malnutrition on later intellectual development (2), I have found that in many of the early studies (e.g., 9,10), the researchers were very careful, in formulating their hypotheses, to try to suggest the pathways by which nutritional insult would influence performance on standardized intelligence tests.

If there is a flaw in most of the studies, it is not the decision to use IQ as an outcome variable, but rather the failure to include in the data analyses other behaviour variables which could be expected, on theoretical grounds, to be influenced by the nutritional variable. The failure to include in one's analyses dependent measures which one would have on theoretical grounds expected to be influenced by the independent variable has been called "restricted generalizability across constructs" (4). The term refers to the fact that the researchers may, by failing to include theoretically relevant outcome variables in their analyses, draw conclusions which are consistent with their data but then incorrectly generalize them to other constructs. For example, in cases where "no significant effect" of malnutrition on IQ were obtained, the researchers might conclude that malnutrition posed no long-term threat to the child's development. However, it might be the case that had more sensitive behavioural indicators of malnutrition been included as dependent variables, effects of malnutrition would have been found. Thus, in our malnutrition research in Guatemala (3,18), we found that early caloric supplementation did not, in general, predict cognitive test performance. However, long-term effects on attention, emotional expression, social involvement and persistence were found. In cases where a significant effect of malnutrition on IQ is identified, failure to include other theoretically relevant outcome variables in data analyses may lead to incorrect inferences about mediating processes (see Barrett (5) for an example).

A final note on IQ testing. IQ tests are samples of behaviour which may be quite powerful as predictors of school performance and general social adjustment (11). In fact, the better tests, and I think that the Wechsler tests (12,13) are the most carefully developed and interpretable, provide an excellent indication of strengths and weaknesses in intellectual ability for preschool to high school age children.

There is no doubt that many researchers have chosen IQ tests as dependent variables for their research because the tests are relatively easy to administer, are widely used, and are accepted as measures of intellectual ability. These are good reasons for using IQ tests to measure intelligence. The more important (i.e., the primary) question is: Is "intelligence" the construct I am interested in as I examine the influence of malnutrition on behaviour? If so, then IQ tests are appropriate dependent measures for the research.

Reaction to the Problem of Reliance on IQ as an Outcome Variable: The "Social Competence Movement"

In recent years there has been a movement to consider "social competence" rather than "IQ" as the criterion for evaluating the effects of intervention programmes for children (and the effects of "risk factors" for later development). There have been three landmark papers. The first was written by Anderson and Messick in 1974 and published in *Developmental Psychology* (14). The second was by Zigler and Trickett in 1978 and published in the *American Psychologist* (15). The third was written by Scarr in 1981 and also published in the *American Psychologist* (16).

Anderson and Messick's paper provided a list of 29 characteristics which were important to consider in studying the development of the child. The list included a number of characteristics in the "social–emotional" domain, for example the child's ability to get along with peers. Zigler and Trickett proposed (15) that "social competence, rather than IQ, should be employed as the major measure of the success of intervention programmes such as Headstart" (p. 793). They defined "social competence" as "emotional/motivational" characteristics including, but not limited to, such characteristics as "effectance motivation", "outerdirectedness and degree of imitation in problem-solving", "positive responsiveness to social reinforcement" and "locus of control". Scarr (16) called for a "new wave of assessments that addresses children's adaptations to situations of interest to the children and the institutions that serve them" (p. 1163). She suggested that intervention studies attempt to measure "the child's motivation and adjustment" (p. 1163).

The reader may detect a note of scepticism in my use of the phrase "social competence movement". Indeed, this shift, this "new wave" movement from "intelligence" to "social competence" as the appropriate criterion for evaluating the child's development represents an advance in one way but a failure in another.

The advance is that it is now well recognized that there are important aspects of child behavioural functioning which are not measured by IQ tests and may be measured in other ways. Researchers concerned with evaluating educational programmes, risk factors for development such as malnutrition or other illness, or rehabilitation for those who have been deprived in some way, no doubt benefit from the knowledge that (a) psychologists and other researchers have conceptualized different dimensions of child behaviour apart from "general intellectual functioning", and (b) these characteristics are measurable and, (c) for some constructs, well developed published tests are available. In the literature on malnutrition research, we now see compendia, listings of variables in different domains and the tests used to measure them. For example, Hurwitz (17) grouped assessment procedures into six categories: Developmental Scales, Tests of General Intelligence, Neuropsychological Test Batteries, Piagetian Scales, Measures of Single Dimensions of Behaviour and Measures of Social–emotional Development. His work provides the researcher a framework for considering not only dimensions of child functioning but also the range of procedures used to measure them.

The *failure* is that the proponents of studying "social competence" often make the same mistake as did those who favoured measuring IQ as an outcome in research. We should not *select* outcome variables as from a catalogue of possible measures. We should *theoretically derive* the variables on the basis of research and theory. Blindly substituting "social competence", "adjustment," "motivation" or a similar construct for "IQ" to fill in the place-holder *y* (dependent variable) in conducting research is just as wrong as blindly accepting IQ as the only dependent variable for a study.

For a dependent variable to be appropriate, two things must hold: (1) we should feel that it is important, that individual differences on the variable have important implications for people, and (2) using the variable should enable us to answer our research question; i.e., the theoretical question.

Next I would like to illustrate the theoretical derivation of constructs for studying the behavioural effects of malnutrition. I will use as an example our research on chronic undernutrition in Guatemala (3,18). Before proceeding there is one question which I would like to briefly address: Can any behaviour be measured?

Can Any Behaviour be Measured?

There are no inherent constraints on what types of behaviours can be reliably measured. As I noted earlier, researchers often fail to measure important dimensions of child behaviour for their research, not because they think them unimportant but because they believe they are too difficult to measure. "Some things just can't be measured," we hear and we begin to believe it's true. But it is not true. If we can think of a characteristic which seems to differentiate people, then there is *nothing* to prevent us from devising a procedure to measure it, that is, to try to document those individual differences. Further, there are no inherent constraints on the reliability and validity, i.e., accuracy and significance,* of measurements obtained using different types of approaches. Reliability and validity are not necessarily better or worse for certain types of procedures (e.g., pencil and paper tests of abilities) than others (e.g., ratings of personality). Reliability and validity are not properties inherent in any single type of measurement procedure. They are characteristics of an instrument which can be *established, worked on* and *improved.* In short, we may greatly underestimate our ability to measure theoretically important aspects of children's behaviour.

Development of Hypotheses and Derivation of Constructs: An Illustration

In research on undernutrition and later behaviour, as in any research, we begin with a hypothesis. The hypothesis makes a formal prediction about the influence of undernutrition on the child's behaviour. Underlying the hypothesis is a theoretical rationale: some notion of the processes whereby such effects might occur. Thus, the research hypothesis should suggest not only the behaviour outcomes which could "ultimately" be affected by the early malnutrition, for example, the school failure or behaviour problems, but also the means by which these outcomes might occur, and, importantly, early behavioural indicators of these developmental problems.

For example, in considering the long-term effects of undernutrition on the child's later intellectual development and social adjustment, we should think about how the experience of undernutrition in infancy might affect the child and family, and how this might influence behaviour. We should also consider how malnutrition continuing after infancy, during a period of rapid social development, might affect the child's peer interactions and experience with the physical environment. By attempting to articulate for ourselves the probable consequences of early nutritional deficit over the course of early

---

* Briefly, reliability is defined as the proportion of variance in a set of observed scores which is "true variance", reflecting true individual differences in the construct of interest rather than "measurement error". The reliability of an instrument is estimated for the instrument for a particular population, and under particular conditions of administration. Thus, an instrument which shows high reliability for one population and under certain conditions of administration may not show high reliability with a different population or under other conditions. Reliability is estimated: it is a theoretical idea. There are many ways to estimate reliability, and all involve obtaining scores on and correlating two administrations of the same test (different forms and/or given at different times) or studying the relationship between parts of the test and the whole (i.e., internal consistency estimates of reliability). The number we obtain is called a reliability coefficient. It is a sample statistic which estimates the true population parameter, that is, the reliability.

The validity of a test, its ability to predict a criterion depends on its reliability. Specifically, if there is a perfectly reliable criterion variable (i.e., theoretically), then the maximum validity for a variable used to predict that criterion is the square root of the reliability. Factors influencing the reliability of a test are given in Magnusson (62).

development, we should be able to develop hypotheses about functional impairments later in childhood and derive dependent variables which represent these outcomes.

In our research, we were concerned with the behavioural effects of chronic undernutrition on the child's social and emotional functioning at school age (3,18). We studied the effects of early caloric supplementation on the behaviour of endemically malnourished children in rural Guatemala.

In beginning to develop hypotheses about the long-term effects on behaviour of chronic undernutrition, we considered two converging lines of research. There are, first, the studies on the behavioural characteristics of malnourished animals, studies which link malnutrition to important functional disorders. Across a variety of species and procedures, severe malnutrition is related to attentional impairments (19), lack of social responsiveness (20,21), emotionality (22,23), avoidance of new stimuli (24), and reduced exploration (21). These findings led us to examine a similar complex of behaviours in human children.

Table 1. Infant studies on behavioural effects of undernutrition.

Investigator	Site	Age at assessment	Behaviour impairment
Lester (25)	Guatemala	1 year	Diminished orienting response
Als *et al.* (26)	USA	first 10 days	Poor motoric processes, low social responsiveness
Brazelton *et al.* (27)	Guatemala	1 month	Poor motoric processes, poor at eliciting social responses, lethargic, difficult to arouse
Mora *et al.* (28)	Colombia	15 days	Irritability
Herrera *et al.* (29)			Poor frustration tolerance; slow visual habituation[a]
Chavez and Martinez (30)	Mexico	1 year	Frequent crying, clinging; high dependency
		18 months	Low activity, infrequent playing
Rush *et al.* (31)	USA	1 year	Short duration of play; slow visual habituation
Zeskind and Ramey (32)	USA	3 years	Withdrawn; anxious[a]
Graves (33,34)	India, Nepal	1–2 years	Reduced exploration

[a] These studies also showed significant effects on measured intelligence at age 3. [b] This table is published in references (3), (38) and (56).

Second, there were recent studies of human infants. Several studies conducted in the last 10 years have attempted to identify dimensions of infant behaviour influenced by prenatal or early postnatal undernutrition. Table 1 shows important studies.

The studies represent two types of research design: one in which growth-retarded infants are compared with normal size infants; the second in which the investigators study the effects of a nutritional supplement given to mothers and/or infants from an endemically malnourished population. The studies give consistent findings and the findings parallel those from the animal research. There ae disturbances in attention, control of emotion, and social responsiveness. Infants with a history of undernutrition have difficulty tolerating frustration, have low activity levels, and lack initiative and independence.

From such studies, we began to develop hypotheses about the behavioural effects of undernutrition by school age. If malnutrition affects attention, responsiveness to social stimuli, and the ability to elicit responses from others, we have the possibility for disruption in caregiver–child interaction. We would expect, based on the "attachment" literature (35–37) that such disturbances would affect the child's behaviour with peers during the toddler and preschool years. Over time, we would expect that the child would learn to withdraw from new situations, would have difficulty in responding to routinely stressful social demands and would lack persistence. In addition we would predict affective withdrawal and reduced physical activity. Table 2 shows predicted behavioural effects of undernutrition at school age.

We decided, then, to measure the following dimensions of the children's social and emotional development at school age: the ability to modulate activity level in different settings and situations, to appropriately express affect, to be socially involved with other children, to respond constructively to moderately stressful problems (such as puzzles, impulse control demands, and competition), to explore new situations and to persist in group activities.

We developed measures of these abilities and refined and construct validated them (3,38). We found strong relationships between the child's early

Table 2. Hypothesized effects of chronic undernutrition at school age.

Infrequent happy affect
Timid or anxious behaviour
Low social involvement
Erratic activity level
Poor impulse control
Poor frustration tolerance
Low exploration
Withdrawal from competitive situations

---

nutritional history, in particular, history of caloric supplementation prenatally and in the first two years, and each of these behaviour characteristics (2,3,18,38).

How Do We Measure?

Once we have decided on the constructs in which we are interested, we have to decide how to operationalize them. I have found it useful to think of measurement in terms of two operations: *data collection* and *data reduction*. Data collection refers to how we collect a sample of behaviour. Data reduction or "coding" refers to how we assign meaning to behaviour.

The methods used for data collection and data reduction should be determined on the basis of psychometric criteria, and in discussing different data collection and data reduction approaches I will discuss these psychometric criteria.

Note, however, that often the data collection method and the data reduction method are implicit in the construct; that is they are defined by our theoretical question. For example, suppose for a particular malnutrition study we are interested in children's aggression. In reviewing the child development research, we find that aggression has been measured in many ways, including frequency of hitting other children, scores on a behaviour checklist for behaviour problems that is filled out by parents, and responses to projective tests. (Each of these methods corresponds to a particular combination of data collection and data reduction methodology. For example, as will be seen from the discussion that follows, the first approach to measuring aggression would correspond to the data collection method "naturalistic observation with time-sampling" and the level of data reduction would be "frequencies".) We might find, further, from reading the publications, that the projective test measure has the highest reported reliability and is the only measure for which validity data were reported.

But suppose our research study has been formulated to provide a test of the theoretical position that, due to their presumed lower activity level, higher inhibition and tendency to withdraw from group activities, early malnourished children are less aggressive to peers than non-malnourished children. In this case we might prefer a behavioural measure of aggression to peers over a projective test of "aggressive character" because it would more closely fit the theoretical construct implicit in the research question.

In the sections that follow, I will discuss the major approaches to data collection and data reduction. Although I have, for this presentation, separated the two procedures, it is important to recognize that, in practice, some of the data collection procedures have certain data reduction or coding methods which tend to "go with them". For example, when one uses *naturalistic observation with time-sampling* to collect data on work or play activities, the behaviours observed are preserved on videotape or film or are immediately translated into behaviour codes by an observer who records the behaviours on paper or calculator. This documentation typically is used to generate *frequency counts* of discrete behaviours, and may allow for scores on *durations* of behaviours. One could also use data collected in this way to generate global *ratings* of subjects' behaviours or code for *presence/absence* of behaviours. Or to take another example, *naturalistic observation with event-sampling* is a data collection method used to collect information about low-frequency events, for example, child comforting of another child crying. Often such data are recorded in a narrative description, and coding usually entails recording the sequences of behaviour acts; e.g., bid for help, followed by comforting response, followed by response to the comforting child. This level of coding I have referred to as *contingent responses*. Conversely, one could use the event-sampling approach to arrive at broad judgements (i.e., *ratings*) about the children in the sample.

Thus, the present separation of data collection from data reduction is made in order to clarify the distinction between how the data are obtained and how they ultimately are assigned meaning but should not be construed as indicating operational independence between the two measurement procedures.

Methods of Data Collection

There are five major categories of data collection in observational behavioural research: (1) naturalistic observation with time-sampling, (2) naturalistic observation with event sampling, (3) experimental situations, (4) naturalistic interventions, and (5) diary records. A sixth category of data collection, standardized tests, is, technically, a type of experimental situation, but I will discuss it separately.

Naturalistic observation with time-sampling

Naturalistic observation is an important method of collecting data in child development research. The essential features are that there are predetermined behaviour categories, that behaviours are sampled over representative situations and over time, and that recording is done "on the spot", whether mechanically or electronically. The strengths of the approach are the possibilities for generating individual scores for rates of behaviour, the generalizability of observations to real-life situations, and the possibility for unobtrusive assessment. An application of this method is given in Barrett *et al.* (18).

Naturalistic observation with event sampling

Often an investigator is interested in a particular behaviour but the behaviour occurs with such low frequency that it is difficult to observe reliably. Or the investigator may wish to describe an episode in detail but may not wish to record all surrounding behaviours. In such cases, a fruitful approach is to observe until a particular type of episode occurs and then to record the specifics of that episode. For example, in the child development research, this approach has been useful in describing the nature of children's aggression and identifying dominance hierarchies in play (39). In the malnutrition research, a version of this approach was used by Nerlove *et al.* (40) in describing the nature of children's day-to-day activities. In this study, on-the-spot, detailed recordings were made of the games and activities of Guatemalan village children and adults, and the episodes later were coded for the content and complexity of the behaviours.

Experimental situations

Major breakthroughs in behavioural research have been made because investigators were able to arrange experimental situations which would allow the subjects to respond to externally imposed manipulations. Much of what we know about children's aggression (41), attachment behaviours (42), and prosocial behaviours (43), as well as the potency of modelling situations (44) has been learned because researchers were ingenious in devising *replicable situations* which might *elicit* or *make possible theoretically important responses.*

In an experimental situation, the investigator has more control over the situation than in naturalistic observation. In fact, the experimental control and the possibility for replication of the observation is the major strength of experimental methodology. Replicability of procedures does not imply reliability of measurements, but it does simplify the training of observers and this may increase the possibility for high interobserver reliability (45).

Experimental situations have been criticized (46) as lacking "generalizability" to real life. However, as Mook has pointed out (47), generalizability does not always have to be a central concern of the researcher. In many studies, what the investigator is trying to do is determine whether a certain condition or treatment could have a certain kind of effect on the organism, and, in order to identify the causal link, attempts to devise a situation that will be as sensitive as possible to the predicted effects. If an experimental situation (or laboratory test) is used to test for this causal effect, it is not necessarily important that behaviour in the experimental test situation generalizes to behaviour in everyday life. What is important is showing how the independent variable *could* affect functioning; i.e. identifying a theoretically predicted causal association.

For example, in the Bogota supplementation study (28), Mora and colleagues predicted that unsupplemented infants would show a stronger emotional response to physical discomfort than supplemented infants. They studied the infant's response to application of a cold disc on the abdomen and found the predicted relationship between nutritional history and response to stress. It was not important whether or not the infant's response to the disc would predict the infant's response to all other types of stress or discomfort. What was important was the identification of a theoretically predicted relationship.

In the malnutrition research, experimental situations have been very useful in showing effects of severe malnutrition on animal behaviour (2). Animal studies examining maze learning, passive and active avoidance responses, and emotional response to stress have involved laboratory experiments. Many of the controlled manipulations in the human research have been embedded in naturalistic situations (see Naturalistic interventions, below). Examples of experimental manipulations are the data collection approaches of Lester (25) studying cardiac habituation of the orienting response in Guatemalan infants; Vuori *et al.* (48) studying visual habituation in the Bogota infants; and Mora *et al.* (28) in the study cited above.

Finally, I would note that laboratory assessments to measure behavioural outcomes are common in other types of nutrition research. For example, much of the research on food additives (e.g., sugar and caffeine) concerns the possible effects on hyperactivity, and thus laboratory measures of attention deficit are often used as dependent variables. The Continuous Performance Test (49) is used in many studies (50,51).

Naturalistic interventions

The strength of experimental testing is replicability. Because the assessment procedures are highly controlled, they can be administered in the same way from one occasion to the next. Experimental assessments may involve, however, disruption of the child's normal activity. This may be a concern not in terms of generalizability, since, as I showed above, generalizability is not always an objective of experimental research, but it may be a concern in that the new situation into which the child is thrust is so strange that a reliable response cannot be made. Thus, it may be useful to embed the situation in a natural context.

Marian Radke-Yarrow and her colleagues (52) demonstrated the utility of this approach in their frequently cited (53) study, "Learning concern for others". The objective was to study influences on children's altruism. But it was critical to obtain large samples of altruistic behaviour and, as those who have observed toddlers or preschool children in daycare or nursery school know, while young children are capable of attending to the physical and emotional needs of others, the frequency of episodes of sharing, comforting and helping in a normal, one-hour play session is very low. The researchers decided to create "prompts" for prosocial intervention. Through a carefully scripted sequence of explicit bids for help, simulations of accidents and problems, and other structured situations, they were able to elicit a wide range of responses to others in need and to generate variables which were reliable and valid.

Examples of naturalistic intervention assessments in nutrition research are Rosenn *et al.*'s stranger approach assessment (55) to study the correlates of failure-to-thrive syndrome, the structured situations (frustration task, response to a novel environment, impulse control situation, competitive game) I used (3) to study the effects of nutritional supplementation on social and emotional functioning in Guatemalan children, and Graves' mother–child interaction situation, used to study the effects of moderate malnutrition on maternal responsiveness and child exploration (33,34).

Diary records

Diary records involve daily recording of child behaviours with a focus on developmental milestones or presence/absence of target (desired or undesired) behaviours. In malnutrition research, diary records have been kept to describe family food practices (i.e., to obtain measurements on the independent variable in the research), but generally have not been used to obtain child behaviour records for use as dependent variables.

A strength of the diary record is unobtrusiveness of measurements. Recording is performed well after the behaviours of interest have occurred. There is no departure from routine and, in fact, the focus is on what occurs during the course of normal, daily activity. Since a major concern of many malnutrition investigations is whether children who have suffered from severe malnutrition in early life are capable of normal development, diary accounts of children's attainments of developmental milestones would appear to be a logical source of outcome date.*

Table 3 summarizes the major strengths of these different data collection approaches.

Standardized tests

Although not often grouped with other behaviour assessment approaches, the approach of standardized testing should be included. Tests, as I said

---

* Problems concerning the reliability and validity of parent reports are discussed in Radke-Yarrow (75).

Table 3. Major strengths of five data collection methods (56).

	TS	ES	EX	NI	DR
Replicability of assessments			*		
Estimates rates of occurrence in real-life situations	*				
Applicable for "low-rate" behaviours		*			
Addresses hypothetical question regarding situational response			*		
Combines features of naturalistic observation (time sampling) and experimental situation				*	
Unobtrusiveness of assessment (with implications for representativeness of behaviour sample)					*

Methods: TS, naturalistic observation with time-sampling; ES, naturalistic observation with event sampling; EX, experimental situations; NI, naturalistic intervention; DR, diary record.

earlier, are experimental situations, controlled manipulations in which the sample of behaviour we obtain is an elicited response to specific stimuli.

Like other experimental situations, standardized tests of intelligence and achievement, such as IQ tests, tests of reading ability, and specialized tests of such abilities as visual memory or discrimination learning, involve highly replicable procedures. The purpose of the test is to discriminate individuals in terms of their responses to these standard situations. The experimental situations are referred to as tests when:

(1) They focus on abilities;
(2) They elicit responses which can be compared to the typical responses of persons in the target population (these data are often published as "norms"); and
(3) Performance involves responses to discrete items or a single task presented in a highly standardized fashion.

Standardized tests of intelligence and achievement are the most widely used measures of behavioural development in the research on the effects of malnutrition on child behaviour. Galler (37) gives a thorough review.

Methods of Data Reduction (Data Coding)

Once a sample of behaviour has been obtained, there are a number of ways in which it can be assigned meaning. The decision about how to code behaviour is primarily one of determining the appropriate "unit of analysis". If we are interested in an infant's affect, do we code each smile and coo, or do we make a more general rating of positive affect? If we are interested in child social adjustment, is it enough to code each child as either well or badly adjusted or should we differentiate children along a continuum?

The major determinant of the appropriate level of analysis is the research objective. What types of causal statements do the investigators hope to be able to make? For example, if the investigator wants to make a statement about improved nutrition and its effects on the rates of certain behaviours, then frequencies have to be scored. If the concern is with mother–child interactive characteristics affected by maternal nutrition, data in the form of contingencies of maternal response to child initiative, or the converse, might be desirable.

There are psychometric considerations. It might seem reasonable, in terms of the investigator's definition of the construct, to operationalize "positive affect" (for example) in terms of number of smiles or happy vocalizations. But it might be that one or both of these variables were difficult to measure reliably. In this case, a different measure would have to be developed.

Six methods for reducing behaviour observations into numerical form are: frequency counts, durations or latencies, ratings (of intensity, frequency or quality of response), proportions of target responses (for behaviours contingent on the occurrence of another behaviour), presence/absence scores, and clinical judgements or classifications.

Frequencies

In many studies, the approach to deriving a score for the child's standing on a variable is to count the number of times the child performs an action. For example, in looking at the effects of malnutrition on sociability (vs. social withdrawal) one might count the number of times the child talks to other children in a set period of time. These behaviours can be converted to rates. Frequencies and rates can be reliable measures if (a) the behaviour to be observed occurs with an adequate frequency, (b) there is agreement among observers about the criteria for what constitutes the behaviour (e.g., are all types of vocalizations "talks"?), and (c) behaviours are observed over sufficient occasions and/or settings so that consistent individual differences will emerge. Epstein (58) showed the importance of "aggregation" of measurements over occasions for reliability.

We used frequency data to describe children's play characteristics in the Guatemala study (18). Few other human studies on the effects of undernutrition have reported frequencies or rates of child behaviours as outcome variables. However, many animal studies, for example studies concerned with "emotionality", have depended on frequency counts to generate their data.

Durations and latencies to respond

Durations of events are often calculated to indicate amount of a characteristic or trait. For example, in malnutrition research, duration of play has been used as a measure of attention (31). When data are preserved on videotape, duration data are likely to be recorded with high reliability, given that the behaviours to be scored (e.g., looks, cries, holds) are clearly defined. Under these conditions, latencies to respond, used, for example, by Mora *et al*. in studying reactivity to aversive stimulation (28) and used also to study impulse control and vigilance, may also be coded with high reliability.

Ratings

Ratings are assignments of values to persons with respect to certain characteristics. The values may represent frequencies, intensities or some other aspect of quality of the variable. Ratings assign the child to a place on a hypothetical continuum, representing that quality.

As I will discuss further in a following section, ratings involve "stepping back from the data" and making judgements, rather than attempting to record precisely what takes place. This "global" aspect of ratings results in certain psychometric strengths but also brings heuristic limitations. I will discuss these in the section "Observations versus Ratings".

Ratings have been frequently used in the malnutrition research. For example, in our study in Guatemala (3,54), children were rated on 1–5 scales, following two days of play and structured activities, on such variables as energy level, work orientation and positive mood. Galler *et al*. (59), in their study in Barbados, had children rated by teachers on attention, obedience, cooperation, memory and distractability. Other variables were coded on a presence/absence basis (see below).

Proportions of target response (contingent responses)

Often we are interested in how a child responds to a particular type of stimulus demand. For example, tests are scored in this way. We look at the proportion of items to which the child responds correctly. With behavioural data, we may wish to examine the child's response to a particular category of antecedent variable, for example, how the child responds to a bid for help or a provocation (60).

In the malnutrition research, DeLicardie and Cravioto (61) used this approach when they attempted to determine whether survivors of early, severe malnutrition responded differently to their own successes and failures (specifically, their "work" or "non-work" responses to demands made by an experimenter) than did children who were not previously malnourished. At Children's Hospital in Boston, we have been conducting a study on the effects of intrauterine growth retardation on the child's development over the first two years of life. I have developed an observation procedure* to study how the mothers respond to their children's involvement with objects; for example, do they encourage the child's exploration or do they try to "redirect" the child's activity. I developed the measure to study maternal responses to infants who might be behaviourally difficult; for example, inattentive and fussy, due to early undernutrition. The procedure involves first identifying infant involvement with a toy (or other activity) and then coding the mother's response to the infant's involvement.

To code at this level of complexity (the level of contingent responses) one must go beyond the subject's behaviour to include, in the behaviour code, the provoking stimulus. When attempting to characterize persons with respect to how they respond to particular cues, one arrives at scores indicating individual differences in proportions of responses having certain characteristics. Individual differences in scores on variables representing behaviours for which either the *response occurs infrequently* or the *antecedent occurs infrequently* are unlikely to have high reliability.

Presence/absence scores

Frequently children will be scored on a variable with respect to whether or not they exhibited a certain characteristic. For example, children may be scored for whether or not they were held back in school, had a criminal record, or had psychiatric problems. Often such measurements can be made very reliably, particularly for variables such as the above which can be agreed upon easily. However, when a continuous distribution is assumed (e.g., for a construct like aggressiveness, patience, helpfulness or assertiveness), ratings of children along the continuum are generally more reliable than forced-choice dichotomies.

Clinical classifications

Classifying persons by making clinical judgements is the most frequently used method for describing the adjustment problems of adults and children receiving psychiatric or psychological treatment. This approach is used also to suggest methods of treatment and the likely effects of treatment. Terms such as schizophrenia, depression and adjustment reaction are terms that most lay people, as well as scientists, recognize as clinical judgements, assigned to persons on the basis of observed behaviours, using techniques such as interviews, tests and real-life observations. Such classifications can be made reliably by trained clinicians (see DSM-III (63), pp. 467–472).

---

* I have written a manual and coding form for this methodology. Descriptions of these materials are available.

Recently, the classification approach has been used to describe individual differences in children in "infant–mother attachment". The construct of attachment comes from Bowlby's (64) interpretation of ethological data on the behaviour of infants of different species toward their parents. Ainsworth and Wittig (65) devised a measurement procedure which they called the "Strange Situation" to study how children respond to separations from the parent, approaches of a stranger, and reunions with the parent, and how they use the parent as a "secure base" for exploration. This method yields classification of children into a group described as "securely attached" and one of two groups described as "insecurely attached". It has been demonstrated (66) that observers can be trained to make such classifications reliably. The distinction between secure and insecure attachments has proved useful in identifying the sequellae of early environmental stresses and predicting later child development outcomes (67). The research of Graves (33,34) and Chavez and Martinez (30) suggests a link between early malnutrition and the development of the infant–mother relationship.

Observations versus Ratings

Cairns and Green (68) showed that the different approaches to assigning meaning to behaviour could be broadly categorized in terms of the distinction of "observations" versus "ratings".

Observations are attempts to record events as they occur. The documentation often takes the form of frequencies, durations, latencies or response contingencies. Scores are usually aggregated across situations, providing summary scores which describe the child's central tendency for the behaviour of interest. For example, if we are looking at a behaviour such as sociability, we might have variables such as rate of social initiation (i.e., frequency per given time interval), average duration of interactions, or proportion of initiations received to which the subject responds with speech.

Ratings are judgements about behaviour, based on but not necessarily describing the specifics of events. The rating is made after the fact. It filters out information that would normally influence the observation but it includes other information. Ratings often are documented as scores on interval scales (e.g., high or low on a five point scale for sociability) or clinical classifications (e.g., depressed).

Cairns and Green point out that the two approaches meet different objectives. The observation approach is sensitive to contextual influences, measuring behaviours which are both situation-general and situation-specific. The rating represents an assessment of the person's enduring behaviour characteristics or traits, one which presumably transcends the specifics of time and place. The rater has the prerogative to selectively use or not use observed events. Thus, given carefully trained raters, ratings are often more predictive than observations, because they are made with the understanding that situational or temporal variations in behaviour are to be overlooked and scores assigned on the basis of what the rater sees as the subject's general response tendencies.

It is clear that the very qualities which make the observation approach attractive in terms of documenting the specifics of events lead to problems in terms of arriving at measures of general traits. Unless one observes across time and setting, generality of observations will be limited. In contrast, the rating approach attempts to more directly estimate individual response tendencies. However, the specifics of behaviours are not preserved, and thus, for some studies, this approach will not address the research question.

In general, I try to use rating methods when (a) I am interested in a construct which is easily understood in terms of our everyday language (e.g., most people would agree on what it means to be involved vs. distracted or to show pleasure vs. lack of pleasure in interaction with others), (b) I have no theoretical interest in trying to differentiate people in terms of their specific acts or interactions but wish to simply estimate the "amount" they have of the attribute in question; and (c) I judge that I will have sufficient time to discuss the construct and its meaning with those who will be carrying out the measurements, agree on operational definitions of the construct, and conduct preliminary reliability analyses to determine whether there is a good chance that the variable will be useful (see footnote on p. 93).

Naturalistic Intervention: An Ilustration from our Research on the Effects of Chronic Undernutrition on Children's Social and Emotional Characteristics

In the previous section I discussed an approach to data collection which I called "Naturalistic Intervention". In the research we conducted in Guatemala on the behavioural effects of early caloric supplementation (3,18,54) we used the naturalistic intervention approach to collect data on important dimensions of emotional functioning. I will discuss the behaviours we were interested in, how we operationalized them, and how we attempted to construct validate them.

In our research we used four different approaches to studying children's behaviour, three of which were based on observations of children in small-group situations. The four types of measurement were (a) measurement of children's responses to particular types of problems and situations in the course of the small-group play activities, (b) measurements of rates of specific behaviours during "free-play" activities in the small groups, (c) ratings made by observers of the children's general behaviour characteristics, following two days of small-group activities, and (d) standardized individual tests of abilities. Here I will be discussing (a), the structured situation measures.

Research Design

I have described in detail (3,18,54) the rationale for the research, the research design, and the results. Briefly, we studied 138 children in rural Guatemala, 78 boys and 60 girls, who had been participants in the INCAP longitudinal study (76). We observed their behaviour when they were ages six to eight years. We examined the relationship between amount of caloric supplementation prenatally and postnatally and behaviour at school age. In the following sections I discuss the measurement of behaviour.

Behaviours of Interest

As I showed earlier, we hypothesized that children with a history of chronic energy deficit would have difficulties, by school age, in responding constructively to routinely stressful challenges and problems. We were interested in studying children's responses to frustration, exploration of a novel environment, impulse control, and response to competition.

General Method for Studying Child Behaviour

We observed children in series of small-group situations. There were six children per group, of the same sex and within one year of age. The age range was six to eight years. We observed 23 groups of children. Observations took place at a central location in the village. Structured tasks were interwoven with free-play activities in two 2½ hour sessions. Observers were experienced Guatemalan observers, all women.

Description of Structured Situations

The structured situations are illustrated in Figs 1a to 1d of reference (3).

First, we looked at the child's response to a novel environment, specifically his/her exploration of a new situation. Children entered a room with novel toys and play materials. We coded for the latency to first contact with a toy, number of materials touched, and the level of involvement with individual toys.

The second situation was a competitive game. It was a relay race played with two teams. Children had to run to the end of a room, pop a balloon with their hands, and run back to touch their team-mate. We were interested in the child's ability to become involved in a physical, exuberant activity and to stay involved in the game. We coded for level of involvement, positive affect, sense of competition and fearfulness about popping the balloons.

The third situation was a frustration task. Children were seated around a table and given a small, clear plastic container with a prize inside. They were told that if they could get the tops off the containers (the tops were almost impossible to pry off) they could get the prize. They were given a small tool, a combination nail-clipper, nail file, to use if they wished. We coded for number of strategies used to solve the problem.

Fourth, we examined motor impulse control. We used a "Simon Says" type game. The experimenter, taking cues from a card behind the children, would say "one-two-three-yes" or "one-two-three-no". The child was directed to clap on "yes" and to refrain from clapping on "no". We coded for number of errors of commission (claps on "no"), errors of omission, and "anticipatory" responses: responses before the command was given.

We predicted that the more undernourished, i.e., the less well-supplemented children, would show the following characteristics. In the unfamiliar situation we predicted less exploration: fewer materials explored and a lower level of involvement. In the group situation involving competition, the prediction was a lower level of participation and greater inhibition, including fearfulness about popping the balloons. In the frustration task, we predicted a tendency to give up easily and to fail to try different strategies. And in the impulse control situation, we expected an inability to inhibit responses (i.e., errors of commission) and also problems sustaining attention (and thus errors of omission).

In addition to the tasks described above, there were two clean-up tasks and a following directions task (where directions were given concerning actions to be carried out following the completion of a task). For each of these situations and for the novel environment situation, degree of initiative in approaching the task was rated on a scale of 1 to 3. The child's average level of initiative across the four situations was computed. We predicted higher scores on initiative for better-supplemented children.

The structured situation measures were, then, as follows:

(1) Novel Environment
    (a) Latency to first contact with toys (rating of 1 to 4)
    (b) Number of materials touched (number from 0 to 5 or more)
    (c) Level of involvement with individual toys (rating of 1 to 3)
(2) Competitive game
    (a) Level of task involvement (rating of 1 to 3)
    (b) Positive affect (rating of 1 to 4)

(c) Sense of competition (presence or absence)

(d) Fearfulness about popping the balloons (rating of 1 to 3)

(3) Frustration Task

(a) Number of strategies used to solve the problem (number from 0 to 7).

(4) Impulse Control Game

(a) Number of errors of commission

(b) Number of errors of omission

(c) Number of anticipatory responses

(5) Initiative

(a) Average rating of initiative (1–3 scale) across three situations.

Evaluating Observer Agreement

To obtain information on observer agreement, two observers watched three (of the six) children per activity. Thus, there were matching observational records. Coefficient "weighted kappa" (69) was computed to determine agreement between raters, correcting for chance agreement. Weighting was linear. Weighted kappas ranged from 0·37 (fearfulness about popping balloons) to 0·95 (sense of competition), with a median of 0·84.

Construct Validation

In any study involving the measurement of behaviour, a major question is whether we are actually measuring what we are trying to measure. This is the problem of construct validity and we address it empirically. Do the behaviours we have measured correlate with, i.e., are they associated with, those behaviours which, by definition of the construct, we expect them to be related to?

In our study, we felt that the structured situations represented the kinds of challenges the child contends with in everyday life. We expected that the different "coping" abilities represented by the different task demands, for example the abilities to cope with frustration and to control impulses, would be closely related. We expected also that children who showed these adaptive capabilities would also be most competent in their peer play. We expected that they would be able to regulate their activity level, show happy affect, and be readily involved with peers.

The relationships between behaviours in the structured situations are illustrated (in a simplified form) in Fig. 1. In this figure, each hexagon represents one of the five types of structured situations: the novel environment ("Exploration"), the competitive game ("Competition"), the frustration task ("Persistence"), the Simons Says game ("Impulse Control") and the tasks of initiative. A line between two hexagons means that for at least one pair of variables measured

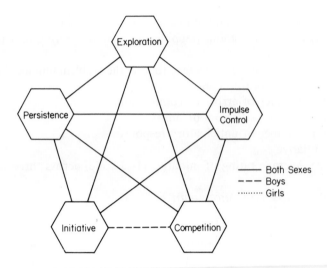

Fig. 1. Associations between children's responses to routinely stressful or challenging situations.

in the situations represented, there was a correlation significant at or below $p < 0.10$. Most such correlations were significant at $p < 0.05$; see (3) and (38).

The method for observing and coding free play with peers has been described (18). Of the many variables we obtained, four were significantly intercorrelated for both boys and girls: happy affect, low anxiety level, high frequency of involvement in the group's activity and moderate activity level.* We found that for each structured situation, at least one measure of responding to that situation was significantly correlated with three or more of these four variables measured in free play.

For example, as shown in Fig. 2, both boys and girls who showed high exploration of the novel environment showed high frequencies of happy

---

* Correlations were:	Boys ($n = 78$)	Girls ($n = 60$)
Happy affect with anxious	$r = -0.57, p < 0.0001$	$r = -0.56, p < 0.0001$
Happy affect with moderate activity level	$r = 0.46, p < 0.0001$	$r = 0.62, p < 0.0001$
Happy affect with involvement in group activity	$r = 0.71, p < 0.0001$	$r = 0.64, p < 0.0001$
Anxious with moderate activity level	$r = -0.70, p < 0.0001$	$r = -0.77, p < 0.0001$
Anxious with involvement in group activity	$r = -0.70, p < 0.0001$	$r = -0.70, p < 0.0001$
Moderate activity level with involvement in group activity	$r = 0.60, p < 0.0001$	$r = 0.86, p < 0.0001$

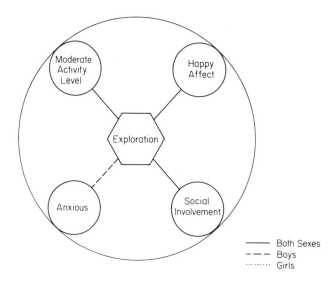

Fig. 2. Associations between exploration in a novel situation and behaviours in free play activities.

affect, moderate activity level, and involvement in the group activity. For boys only, exploration was also associated with low scores on anxiety.

In sum, children, who were competent in the structured situations were also competent with peers in free play. Complete tables of correlations are given in (3) and (38), and figures illustrating the associations appear in (56).

Effects of Undernutrition

The results of this study have already been reported (3,18,54). The results confirmed our hypotheses about the effects of early nutritional supplementation on children's later behaviour. On structured situations, high-supplemented children had higher scores than low-supplemented children on Number of Materials Touched and Level of Involvement with toys in the Novel Environment, scored higher on Level of Task Involvement in the Competitive Game, and used more strategies on the Frustration Task, and made fewer errors of omission in the Impulse Control Game. Predicted effects of nutritional supplementation on behaviours in peer play, reported in (18), were also obtained.

The Importance of an Explicity Developmental Framework for Formulating Behavioural Measures for Research on Effects of Malnutrition

I would like to close by discussing the importance of an understanding of child development for the development of measures of children's behaviour. Specifically, the importance of knowing what behaviours are important at different times in the child's development.

There are certain aspects of child behaviour which can be reliably observed only at certain ages, since these behaviours represent "tasks" which the child is trying to master at those ages. For example, in studying the effects of a nutritional variable on child exploration, we must conceptualize exploration differently at different ages. At age four months we can think about the child's interest in reaching for and grasping objects. At nine months we can attempt to measure the child's interest in creating stimulation by his/her own locomotion; for example, by crawling toward interesting objects. At 12 months when the child is interested in exploring the properties of objects (in/on; on top/under; contains/doesn't contain) we can study individual differences in their interest in and exploration of these properties. And at 18 to 24 months, with the child's developing self-awareness (70), we can look at the child's exploration of himself in relation to the object world: for example, his interest in attempting new problems, his inhibition in the face of novel stimuli, and his persistence when challenged.

When we use our understanding of "developmental tasks" to formulate behaviour variables, we are likely to generate reliable assessments, since we will be attempting to estimate true variance in behaviours on which there are true individual differences. If we fail to consider developmental changes in the importance of different behaviours, our measurements will not be reliable. For example, to use the illustration I just discussed, if an investigator wishes to study the effects of malnutrition on exploration of toys at three months, he will fail to detect reliable individual differences in the exploration variable because the child is more interested in face-to-face interaction with the mother, with mutual smiling and vocalizing. However, if the investigator is interested in differences in child smiling to the mother's face in face-to-face interaction, if he measures at five months he will fail to detect reliable differences because the child will be starting to "break away" from the mother and trying to look at and reach for objects.

Similarly, studies of the effects of malnutrition on infant–mother attachment (i.e., response to the mother's leaving and then returning in the Ainsworth Strange Situation) should be done at about age one year and before 18 months. Why? Because as the child approaches two years he will begin to better understand that the mother can go away for a short time and not be permanently lost. The reunion test will thus lose its potency as a measure of the child's "security of attachment". The reason the test is so potent at one year is that even though the child has attained a certain level of object permanence (he will consistently search for a hidden object) he has not yet attained that level of object understanding that he *knows* that if a person leaves a room they must be somewhere else, that they continue to exist in that new place, and that they can return to the original place. The child's understanding of object permanence is still uncertain.

One of the reasons this understanding of development is so important is that we are now seeing an interest in studying the effects of malnutrition on mother–child interaction in infancy (71). From the first reports of behavioural effects of undernutrition in infancy (72) there has been a recognition that early protein–calorie malnutrition affects the behaviour of the infant and may alter the course of the mother–child relationship (73), particularly when the mother may also be malnourished. The failure-to-thrive literature (74) has been particularly concerned with undernutrition in the context of an impoverished environment as it affects the mother–infant dyad. Several have suggested that changes in the mother–infant relationship mediate the relationship between early undernutrition and later child behaviour problems (18).

In measuring maternal behaviour towards the child as an outcome of undernutrition and a possible means by which the child's behavioural development can be impaired, it is *critical* that we first try to understand what the child's developmental task or tasks are in the time period of interest. We will then be able to formulate and construct reliable and meaningful maternal behaviour variables.

For example, one of the problems I see among researchers trying to study maternal behaviour as an outcome variable is that there is a tendency to underestimate the importance of the mother's allowing the child to explore the environment. Most researchers have tended to conceptualize "maternal responsiveness" in terms of affection and nurturance. Specifically, there has been a tendency to look for maternal behaviours with infants of five months and older which would be more appropriate with the child of two to three months. One of the things I try to point out to researchers who are studying parent–infant interaction is that the parent's "tasks" change dramatically at about four to five months because of changes in the child's interests and abilities. When the child is two to three months old, he is content to sit in an infant seat looking at his mother and father and to engage in long, back and forth exchanges of smiling and vocalizing. A "responsive mother" for the child this age is one who responds in a reciprocal manner to the child's looks, smiles and cooing. But by age four to five months, most infants will not even sit still for a long time in an infant seat. They squirm around, try to get out, and are more interested in reaching for objects around them than in looking at the mother's face. The "responsive mother" at this age pays attention to and supports her baby's new interest in and understanding of the object world. She laughs and smiles at his antics but also allows him to look away, "giving him room" to attend to the objects he is interested in. A mother who keeps trying to engage the baby in face-to-face interaction at this age is probably being intrusive rather than "responsive".

In sum, understanding the child's development — his developing interests, abilities and needs–is necessary if we are to formulate meaningful outcome variables for research on malnutrition and behaviour. It is particularly important when our outcomes focus on the mother's ability to respond appropriately to the child's needs.

Summary

In this paper I have attempted to make the following points.

(1) Any behaviour can be measured. When we determine outcome variables for research on malnutrition and behaviour, we should theoretically derive them, and not select them on atheoretical grounds. Recently, there has been a shift in interest from cognitive to "social–emotional" variables as outcome variables for malnutrition. This is fine as long as we choose our variables (whether cognitive or social–emotional) on theoretical grounds. What we should not be doing is saying: "Now here is a list of all the types of social and emotional characteristics one could conceivably measure. Which ones should we choose?"

(2) Once the appropriate *construct* has been derived for study, we can operationalize it in many ways. The two processes in measurement are data collection and data reduction. I described six approaches to data collection and their strengths and limitations for different research purposes. I discussed six "levels" of data reduction, contrasting, in particular, the psychometric properties of ratings versus observations (e.g., frequency counts). Both data collection and data reduction procedures must be based primarily on theoretical considerations. That is, we try to make the operational definition of the variable "fit" the theoretical conceptualization.

(3) In our research, we have been able to develop reliable and valid measures of children's emotional characteristics at school age, using an approach called "naturalistic intervention". This involves "perturbing" the child's natural play activities to better elicit behaviours of interest. On the basis of previous malnutrition research,

we had hypothesized long-term effects of early caloric deficit (and supplementation) on the child's ability to deal constructively with moderately stressful problems. We used the naturalistic intervention approach to collect data on children's responses to novel, frustrating and competitive situations. We construct validated the measures by studying the relationships between these situational measures and theoretically relevant aspects of "free play" with peers. We found significant effects of early caloric undernutrition (specifically, high or low supplementation) and these measures of child response to stressful situations.

(4) In developing behavioural measures for malnutrition research, it is critical that we do so from a developmental framework. If we are studying children at one year, we should be thinking of the developmental "tasks" of the one-year-old. If we are concerned with maternal behaviour toward the undernourished four-month-old, we should be thinking about the developmental needs of the four-month-old and his parents. If, as we formulate behaviour variables, we fail to consider the developmental level of the child, his interests and needs, the variables we generate are unlikely to be useful.

References

1. Levine, S. and Wiener, S. (1976). A critical analysis of data on malnutrition and behavioral deficits. *Adv. Pediat.* **22**, 113–136.
2. Barrett, D. E. and Frank, D. A. (1987). "The Effects of Undernutrition on Children's Behavior." Gordon and Breach, New York.
3. Barrett, D. E. and Radke-Yarrow, M. R. (1985). Effects of nutritional supplementation on children's responses to novel, frustrating and competitive situations. *Am. J. Clin. Nutr.* **42**, 102–120.
4. Cook, T. D. and Campbell, D. T. (1979). D. T. "Quasi-experimentation: Design and Analysis Issues for Field Settings." Rand-McNally, Chicago.
5. Barrett, D. E. (1984). Methodological requirements for conceptually valid research studies on the behavioral effects of malnutrition. *In* "Nutrition and Behavior" (J. R. Galler, ed.) pp. 9–36. Plenum Press, New York.
6. Lloyd-Still, J. D. (1976). Clinical studies on the effects of malnutrition during infancy on subsequent physical and intellectual development. *In* "Malnutrition and Mental Development" (J. D. Lloyd-Still, ed.) pp. 103–159. Publishing Sciences Group, Littleton, MA.
7. Pollitt, E. and Thomson, C. (1977). Protein–calorie malnutrition and behavior: a view from psychology. *In* "Nutrition and the Brain" (R. J. Wurtman and J. J. Wurtman, eds) Vol. 2, pp. 261–306. Basic Books, New York.
8. Brožek, J. (1977). Nutrition, malnutrition and behavior. *Ann. Rev. Psychol.* **29**, 157–177.
9. Evans, D., Moodie, A. D. and Hansen, J. D. L. (1971). Kwashiorkor and intellectual development. *S. Afr. Med. J.* **45**, 1414–1426.

10. Hertzig, M. E., Birch, H. G., Richardson, S. A. and Tizard, J. (1972). Intellectual levels of school children severely malnourished during the first two years of life. *Pediat.* **49**, 814–824.

11. Sattler, J. M. (1982). "Assessment of Children's Intelligence and Special Abilities", 2nd edn. Allyn and Bacon, Boston.

12. Wechsler, D. (1974). "Manual for the Wechsler Intelligence Scale for Children — Revised." Psychological Corporation, New York.

13. Wechsler, D. (1967). "Manual for the Wechsler Preschool and Primary Scale of Intelligence." Psychological Corporation, New York.

14. Anderson, S. and Messick, S. (1974). Social competence in young children. *Devl. Psychol.* **10**, 282–293.

15. Zigler, E. and Trickett, P. K. (1978). IQ, social competence, and evaluation of early childhood intervention programs. *Am. Psychol.* **33**, 789–798.

16. Scarr, S. (1981). Testing *for* children: Assessment and the many determinants of intellectual competence. *Am. Psychol.* **36**, 1159–1166.

17. Hurwitz, I. Psychometric methods. *In* "Malnutrition and Behavior: A Critical Assessment of Key Issues" (J. Brožek and B. Schürch, eds) pp. 164–176. Nestlé Foundation, Lausanne, Switzerland.

18. Barrett, D. E., Radke-Yarrow, M. and Klein, R. E. (1982). Chronic malnutrition and child behavior: Effects of early caloric supplementation on social-emotional functioning at school age. *Devl. Psychol.* **18**, 541–556.

19. Zimmerman, R. R., Geist, C. R., Strobel, D. A. and Cleveland, T. J. (1974). Attention deficits in malnourished monkeys. *In* "Early Malnutrition and Mental Development" (J. Cravioto, L. Hambraeus and B. Vahlquist, eds) pp. 115–126. Almquist and Wiksell, Uppsala, Sweden.

20. Zimmerman, R. R., Steere, P. O., Strobel, D. A. and Hom, H. L. (1972). Abnormal social development of protein malnourished monkeys. *J. Abnorm. Psychol.* **80**, 125–131.

21. Fraňková, S. (1973). Effect of protein–calories malnutrition on the development of social behavior in rats. *Devl. Psychobiol.* **6**, 33–43.

22. Fraňková, S. and Barnes, R. H. (1968). Effect of malnutrition in early life on avoidance conditioning and behavior of adult rats. *J. Nutr.* **96**, 486–493.

23. Barnes, R. H., Moore, A. U. and Pond, W. G. (1970). Behavioral abnormalities in young adult pigs caused by malnutrition in early life. *J. Nutr.* **100**, 149–155.

24. Strobel, D. A. and Zimmerman, R. R. (1972). Responsiveness of protein-deficient monkeys to manipulative stimuli. *Devl. Psychobiol.* **5**, 291–296.

25. Lester, B. M. (1975). Cardiac habituation of the orienting response in infants of varying nutritional status. *Devl. Psychol.* **11**, 432–442.

26. Als, H., Tronick, E., Adamson L. and Brazelton, T. B. (1976). The behavior of the underweight but full-term newborn infant. *Dev. Med. Child. Neurol.* **18**, 590–602.

27. Brazelton, T. B., Tronick, E., Lechtig, A., Lasky, R. E. and Klein, R. E. (1977). The behavior of nutritionally deprived Guatemalan infants. *Dev. Med. Child. Neurol.* **19**, 364–372.

28. Mora, J. O., Clement, J., Christiansen, N., Ortiz, N., Vuori, L. and Wagner, M. (1979). Nutritional supplementation, early stimulation and child development. *In* "Proceedings of an International Conference on Energy and Protein Deficits" (J. Brožek, ed.) pp. 255–268. DHEW (NIH), Washington, DC.

29. Herrera, M. G., Mora, J. O., Christiansen, N., Ortiz, N., Clement, J., Vuori, L., Waber, D., De Paredes, B. and Wagner, M. (1980). Effects of nutritional

supplementation and early education on physical and cognitive development. *In* "Life-Span Developmental Psychology" (R. R. Turner and F. Reese, eds) pp. 149–184. Academic Press, New York.

30. Chavez, A. and Martinez, C. (1979). Consequences of insufficient nutrition on character and behavior. *In* "Malnutrition, Environment, and Behavior" (D. A. Levitsky, ed.) pp. 238–268. Cornell University Press, Ithaca, NY.

31. Rush, D. S., Stein, Z. and Susser, M. (1980). A randomized control trial of prenatal nutritional supplementation in New York City. *Pediat.* **65**, 683–697.

32. Zeskind, P. S. and Ramey, C. T. (1981). Preventing intellectual and interactional sequelae of fetal malnutrition: a longitudinal, transactional, and synergistic approach to development. *Child Dev.* **52**, 213–218.

33. Graves, P. L. (1976). Nutrition, infant behavior, and maternal characteristics: a pilot study in West Bengal, India. *Am. J. Clin. Nutr.* **29**, 305–319.

34. Graves, P. L. (1978). Nutrition and infant behavior: a replication study in the Katmandu Valley, Nepal. *Am. J. Clin. Nutr.* **31**, 541–555.

35. Lieberman, A. F. (1977). Preschoolers' competence with a peer: relations with attachment and peer experience. *Child Dev.* **48**, 1277–1287.

36. Easterbrooks, M. A. and Lamb, M. E. (1979). The relationship between the quality of mother–infant attachment and infant competence in initial encounters with peers. *Child Dev.* **50**, 380–387.

37. Waters, E., Wippman, J. and Sroufe, L. A. (1979). Attachment, positive affect the competence in the peer group: two studies in construct validation. *Child Dev.* **50**, 821–829.

38. Barrett, D. E. (1986). Nutrition and social behavior. *In* "Theory and Research in Behavioral Pediatrics" (H. E. Fitzgerald, B. M. Lester and M. W. Yogman, eds) Vol. 3, pp. 147–198. Plenum Press, New York.

39. Strayer, F. G. and Strayer, J. (1976). An ethological analysis of social agonism and dominance relations among preschool children. *Child Dev.* **47**, 980–989.

40. Nerlove, S. B., Roberts, J. M., Klein, R. E., Yarbrough, C. and Habicht, J. P. (1974). Natural indicators of cognitive development: an observational study of rural Guatemalan children. *Ethos.* **2**, 265–295.

41. Liebert, R. M. and Baron, R. A. (1972). Some immediate effects of televised violence on children's behavior. *Devl. Psychol.* **6**, 469–475.

42. Ainsworth, M. D. S., Blehar, M. C., Waters, E. and Wall, S. (1978). "Patterns of Attachment: A Psychological Study of the Strange Situation." Lawrence Erlbaum, Hillsdale, NJ.

43. Staub, E. (1978). "Positive Social Behavior and Morality", Vol. I. Academic Press, New York.

44. Bandura, A., Ross, D. and Ross, S. (1961). Transmission of aggression through imitation of aggressive models. *J. Abn. Soc. Psychol.* **63**, 375–382.

45. Johnson, S. M. and Bolstad, O. D. (1973). Methodological issues in naturalistic observation: some problems and solutions for field research. *In* "Behavior Change: Methodology, Concepts and Practice" (L. A. Hamerlynck, L. C. Handy and E. J. Mash, eds) pp. 1–67. Research Press, Champaign, Illinois.

46. Babbie, E. R. (1975). "The Practice of Social Science Research." Wadsworth, Belmont, CA.

47. Mook, D. (1983). In defense of external invalidity. *Am. Psychol.* **38**, 379–387.

48. Vuori, L., de Vavarro, L., Christiansen, N., Mora, J. O., Wagner, M. and Herrera, M. G. (1979). Nutritional supplementation and the outcome of pregnancy. II. Visual habituation at 15 days. *Am. J. Clin. Nutr.* **32**, 463–469.

49. Rosvold, H., Mirsky, A., Sarason, I., Bransome, E. J., Jr and Beck, L. H. (1956). A continuous performance test of brain damage. *J. Consult. Psychol.* **20**, 343–350.
50. Ferguson, H. B., Stoddart, C. and Simeon, J. G. (1986). Double-blind challenge studies of behavioral and cognitive effects of sucrose-aspertame ingestion in normal children. *Nutr. Rev. Suppl.* **44**, 144–150.
51. Prinz, R. J. and Riddle, D. B. (1986). Associations between nutrition and behavior in 5-year-old children. *Nutr. Rev. Suppl.* **44**, 151–158.
52. Yarrow, M. R., Scott, P. M. and Waxler, C. Z. (1973). Learning concern for others. *Devl. Psychol.* **8**, 240–260.
53. Mussen, P. M. and Eisenberg-Berg, N. (1978). "Roots of Caring, Sharing and Helping." Jossey-Bass, San Francisco.
54. Barrett, D. E. (1984). Malnutrition and child behavior: conceptualization, assessment and an empirical study of social–emotional functioning. *In* "Malnutrition and Behavior: A Critical Assessment of Key Issues" (J. Brožek and B. Schürch, eds) pp. 280–306. Nestlé Foundation, Lausanne, Switzerland.
55. Rosenn, D., Loeb, L. and Jura, M. (1980). Differentiation of organic from non-organic failure-to-thrive syndrome in infancy. *Pediat.* **66**, 698–704.
56. Barrett, D. E. (1986). Behavior as an outcome in nutrition research. *Nutr. Rev. Suppl.* **44**, 224–236.
57. Galler, J. R. (1984). The behavioral consequences of malnutrition in early life. *In* "Nutrition and Behavior," (J. R. Galler, ed.) pp. 63–117. Plenum Press, New York.
58. Epstein, S. (1980). The stability of behavior. II. Implications for psychological research. *Am. Psychol.* **35**, 790–808.
59. Galler, J. R., Ramsey, F., Solimano, G. and Lowell, W. E. (1983). The influence of early malnutrition on subsequent behavioral development. II. Classroom behavior. *J. Am. Acad. Child. Psychiatry.* **22**, 16–22.
60. Barrett, D. E. (1979). A naturalistic study of sex differences in children's aggression. *Merrill-Palmer Quarterly* **25**, 193–203.
61. DeLicardie, E. R. and Cravioto, J. (1974). Behavioral responsiveness of survivors of clinically severe malnutrition to cognitive demands. *In* "Early Malnutrition and Mental Development" (J. Cravioto, L. Hambraeus and B. Vahlquist, eds) pp. 134–154. Almquist and Wiksell, Uppsala, Sweden.
62. Magnussen, D. (1966). "Test Theory". Addison-Wesley, Reading, MA.
63. "Diagnostic and Statistical Manual of Mental Disorders", 3rd edn (1980). American Psychiatric Association, Washington DC.
64. Bowlby, J. (1958). The nature of the child's tie to his mother. *Int. J. Psychoanal.* **39**, 350–373.
65. Ainsworth, M. and Wittig, B. (1969). Attachment and exploratory behavior in one-year-olds in a strange situation. *In* "Determinants of Infant Behavior" (B. Foss, ed.) Vol. 4, pp. 111–136. Methuen, London.
66. Waters, E. (1978). The reliability and stability of individual differences in infant–mother attachment. *Child Dev.* **49**, 483–494.
67. Lewis, M., Feiring, C., McGuffog, C. and Jaskir, J. (1984). Predicting psychopathology in six-year-olds from early social relations. *Child Dev.* **55**, 123–136.
68. Cairns, R. B. and Green, J. A. (1979). How to assess personality and social patterns: observations or ratings? *In* "The Analysis of Social Interactions" (R. B. Cairns, ed.) pp. 209–226. Lawrence Erlbaum, Hillsdale, NJ.

69. Cohen, J. (1968). Weighted kappa: nominal scale agreement with provision for scaled disagreement or partial credit. *Psychol. Bull.* **70**, 213–220.
70. Kagan, J. (1982). The emergence of self. *J. Child Psychol. Psychiatry.* **23**, 363–381.
71. Galler, J. R., Ricciuiti, H. N., Crawford, M. A. and Jucharski, L. T. (1984). The role of the mother–infant interaction in nutritional disorders. *In* "Nutrition and Behavior" (J. R. Galler, ed.) pp. 269–304. Plenum Press, New York.
72. Geber, M. and Dean, R. (1956). The psychological changes accompanying kwashiorkor. *Courrier.* **6**, 3–14.
73. Lester, B. M. (1979). A synergistic process approach to the study of prenatal malnutrition. *Int. J. Behav. Devel* **2**, 377–394.
74. Frank, D. A. (1984). Malnutrition and child behavior: a view from the bedside. *In* "Malnutrition and Behavior: A Critical Assessment of Key Issue" (J. Brožek and B. Schürch, eds) pp. 307–326. Nestlé Foundation, Lausanne, Switzerland.
75. Radke-Yarrow, M. (1963). Problems of methods in parent–child research. *Child Devel.* **34**, 215–226.
76. Klein, R. E., Irwin, M., Engle, P. L. and Yarbrough, C. (1977). Malnutrition and mental development in rural Guatemala. *In* "Studies in Cross-cultural Psychology" (N. Warren, ed.) pp. 91–119. Academic Press, New York.

Commentary

J. L. Smart: Barrett's investigation of the effects of undernutrition on "social competence" was long overdue.

My first comment is on methodology and may well be answered in more detailed accounts of Barrett's study in Guatemala. It relates to the composition of the groups of six children. We are told that they were of the same sex and within one year of age, but not about the nutritional history of the members or whether they knew one another before being grouped for the study. Were efforts made to group together children with the same or with different nutritional histories or was this factor and previous acquaintanceship left to chance or randomized in the creation of the groups?

A more general point relates to Barrett's insistence that outcome variables should be theoretically derived; that is, that choice of what to measure or score should be on theoretical grounds. No-one could do other than applaud this recommendation, at least in principle. It is only when I examine it in the light of my experience of my own and others' research and subject this to frank appraisal that the recommendation wears thin.

The desire for a theoretical basis no doubt stems from the Physical Sciences where the progression from existing knowledge to theory to hypothesis to experiment is the *sine qua non* of good practice. The psychologist earnestly hopes that by adopting the framework of the hard physical sciences he will render his soft science more firm. This is fine in principle, but it does rather fall down when one realizes that in much of psychology the "existing knowledge", which is the starting point for the logical sequence, is so soft as to render subsequent theorizing very questionable. So perhaps one ought to admit that there are different levels of theoretical derivation. That used by Barrett does not seem to be a high level: which is not a criticism but an observation, since that was probably all that was available to him. This kind of derivation is probably better thought of as extrapolation rather than theory. Furthermore, part of it is based on conclusions from a selective and personal review of the animal undernutrition literature, which would differ in some respects from my conclusions and those of other reviewers.

But does it matter? No matter how derived, Barrett arrives at an "hypothesis" or set of "hypotheses" which form the bases for his observational studies. The findings are fascinating. No, at this level of theorizing it does not matter, since it is hardly theorizing at all. It would matter, I think, if any hypothesis regarding mechanisms were derived from theory. Then, if the theorizing were flawed, the conclusions regarding the mechanism would be likely also to be flawed.

Perhaps we researchers should come clean and admit to ourselves and others that our "hypotheses" (if that is not too grand a term) are sometimes derived from "feelings" about our subjects, be they animal or human. We feel, based on casual observation, that they differ in such-and-such a way from normal. This is not unscientific: it is a progression from casual observation, or, if you prefer, pilot study, to hypothesis to definitive study. This seems to me perfectly valid and, if not as intellectually satisfying as aping the physical sciences, more honest than pretending to do so in many cases.

I. Hurwitz: Barrett provides systematic presentation of the structure of a research enterprise from its conceptual inception to its eventual implementation and interpretation. One may say that this paper could be profitably used in an educational setting to demonstrate to students the sequential process by which research efforts come into existence. While the focus obviously is on investigative efforts in the field of undernutrition, this contribution provides a model for a broad spectrum of studies in which the issue is the assessment of an intervention programme applied to populations of varied interest to the scientific community and investigator, whether it be nutrition, family divorce, abuse, separation, etc. Barrett de-mystifies the confusion surrounding much of what has appeared to be the critical stumbling blocks in the development of research efforts in the specific fields of nutritional studies, namely, the clear and concise definitions of terms such as construct, variable, measurement, etc. as these apply to this particular field. There is an unmistakable quality of refreshing clarity in Barrett's efforts to present us with this catalogue of relevant research issues. However, what perhaps should have been most energetically emphasized in Barrett's opening section and yet seems underplayed, is the crucial importance of theory itself as the basis from which the variety of factors designated as independent variables are ultimately derived. It is not entirely clear what Barrett means by theory in this context, i.e., whether he looks to a broad theory of cognitive and/or social development which can then be integrated with a theory of biological development and which in turn can generate hypotheses which are comprehensive and biopsychological in nature, encompassing both dimensions. For example, one may consider a Piagetian view of development on the one hand with its emphasis on stage-related phenomena as encompassing the emergence of one set of consequences in the face of early undernutrition, namely deficits in cognitive phenomena, and on the other hand a neurobiological theory of critical periods of central nervous system development which serves as the substrate for these cognitive processes. Based on these two theoretical frames of reference, it may be possible to formulate hypotheses which can then be subjected to experimental verification through the selection of appropriate procedures from any of the various measurements approaches which Barrett outlines, or which may be taken from other sources including Dasen's work on Piagetian techniques in malnutrition studies, or the work of Pinard and Laurendeau in the field of spatial concepts and causal thinking. Biological variables of course emanate from the use of animal models as defined in the paper contributed to this volume by Smart and the studies reported by Bedi. However, in the Guatemalan study described here, Barrett chooses, one might say, to formulate a theory based on the developmental origins of social behaviour, though even here one sees less of a "theory" than a collection of empirical findings effectively "reduced" to broader psychological categories such as attention, cooperation, impulsiveness, etc. and tied to a variety of operational definitions which have translated into measuring techniques ranging from time sampling to psychometric assessment. Still, there is no question but what the methodological characteristics of Barrett's Guatemala study are far reaching and important in scope and implications. They make possible a far clearer grasp of the multiple corrosive inroads into adequate cognitive and social behaviours which malnutrition and undernutrition bring about, and in addition supply a model of reasonable technical tactics for further research. The caveat supplied by Barrett at the close of the report with respect to understanding developmental changes in social behaviour at different time points is of vital significance, as is the obligatory reference he makes to cross-cultural factors which must be taken into account in any relevant design.

This paper, despite its enormous value, still leaves one with the dual task of *creating* theory and, with such theory, developing a method of research investigation which sensibly adheres to what Luria once referred to as "restrictive sampling", i.e., assessing those areas of behaviour which are most productive in their yield of data expanding our knowledge in the chosen field of endeavour.

Author's reply: I am referring by "theory" to a set of constructs, interrelated by means of propositions and extrapolations, which is generally understood by scientists in a given field as generating testable hypotheses about phenomena of interest. This set of constructs or "theoretical framework" may include constructs which have been formulated on the basis of different types of observation and theory. For example the same theoretical framework attempting to account for individual differences in child competence on the basis of early nutritional history may include constructs such as "functional isolation" derived empirically from the experimental animal research, and constructs such as "attachment", derived both from ethological studies of animals and clinical observations of mothers and infants.

S. A. Richardson: The paper focusses on how to measure the behaviour of children. This is a useful review, but I would like to have seen the addition of sections dealing with the use of interviews, documentary sources, sociometry and longitudinal measures.

Throughout the review there appears to be an implicit assumption that the early nutritional status of the child is the variable which accounts for the differences found later in children's behaviour.

There is general agreement that children with an early history of undernutrition later function less well than children with adequate early nutrition. To me the major question is what factors may account for this difference. In the studies that have addressed this question it is clear that the measurement of undernutrition and the measurements of children's environmental experiences are the major problems which have received relatively little attention compared to measures of the individual child. I would have liked to have seen a paper dealing with how to measure environmental factors that directly and indirectly interact with children using a longitudinal and ecological perspective.

J. Dobbing: Barrett makes the point that we should not merely select the behavioural outcomes as from a catalogue when we want to measure the results of early undernutrition on behaviour, and I take his point. However many of us are really asking a question which is no more specific than "Does malnutrition in early life specifically lead to deleterious effects on those parts of behaviour which we, as humans, particularly value, and which are often our most distinguishing characteristics?''. In other words we are prepared to be fairly specific about "malnutrition", amongst all the other factors in the environment which affect our later behaviour, but we do not know what behaviour we are asking about except that it should *matter*. We are not even sure that nutrition has *any* such effect. The technology of developmental behavioural science is not our personal interest, except in so far as we want to have it used reputably. In a sense this is the attitude of the ordinary citizen rather than of the scientist, but can those of us who are not behavioural scientists do any different?

Therefore it seems to me, at least in these early stages of the enquiry, that a catalogue, or a trawl, may not (*exceptionally*) be such a bad idea, as long as proper investigations are designed and proper techniques used. Against the fashion, I am not convinced that the "look and see" approach, provided it is disciplined and technically sound, is always a bad thing, again in these early stages.

I am not confident that it is so wrong to say that "Some things just can't be measured''. Certainly there are things which we know to be valuable which are barely definable, and can therefore not be measured until they are, but that does not make them reprehensible in science. Science is about taking everything into account, and many of the wider aspects of natural science seem to me to be in this hard-to-define category. Perhaps Barrett is only against the idea of saying that "Some things will never be measurable''; but that is another matter. He may well be able to define "death"; or "love"; or even "emotion"; but it will only be *his* definition and not necessarily the article we are interested in, however conveniently it may fit into an experimental protocol!

I cannot see that proper design of all investigations demands that we should always postulate a mechanism for any effect we are looking for. I can, for example, try out a treatment for a disease without having the first idea how it might work; and the epidemiologist can look for associations without any notion about the possible correlative pathway. Even though this latter example can lead sometimes to epidemiological rubbish, I think that it is often a *better* strategy in applied science to look first for your phenomenon and get it established (are undernourished children *for that reason* in any way disadvantaged in later life?) before researching the possible mechanisms by which it may be so. The latter approach has led biochemists, for example, and perhaps even behavioural scientists, up many garden paths of less useful self-generated research.

I notice that all the supposed animal analogies mentioned as inspirational for research into our subject date from 1968–73. We have moved on since then, and many of these papers, and hence their inspirational power, would probably be seriously flawed today.

I can find next to no question in this paper about the specific effects on behaviour of nutrition as a component of a complex environment, nor any attempt to measure its effects relative to all the other factors. And that is one of the more important questions.

K. S. Bedi: One of the things that worries me slightly is the great reliance that Barrett places on tests of correlation. These are usually fairly "weak" statistical tests. It is all too easy to get statistically significant correlations between otherwise completely unrelated things.

The "kappa" scores used to evaluate observer agreement are also slightly worrying. Does a score of $0 \cdot 37$ indicate that there was not very good agreement between observers of the same task?

Author's reply: Bedi says that correlation coefficients are "weak statistical tests". They are no less powerful than t-tests or the analysis of variance. It is true that they do not necessarily demonstrate causation. However, they are nevertheless useful for identifying scientific relations. Correlational analyses, carefully conceived on the basis of theory and prior research and carefully interpreted, may be very important in contributing to our understanding of possible causal influences on outcomes of interest.

The kappa coefficient referred to ($0 \cdot 37$) was statistically significant; that is there was a higher-than-chance level of agreement between observers. However, a kappa of $0 \cdot 37$ is not high. It shows a relatively high level of disagreement between observers, and as an indicator of reliability (or unreliability), suggests that the variable being measured is not being measured with a high degree of precision.

D. A. Levitsky and Barbara J. Strupp. The focus of Barrett's paper is the development of sensitive indicators of the subtle effects of poor nutrition (and of other insults) on the behaviour of children. The emphasis that Barrett places on designing the measurements of behaviour on sound theoretical deductions rather than choosing conventional measures, such as IQ or school grades, cannot be overemphasized.

However, in all fairness to the majority of large-scale studies that have used "Standard Intelligence Tests" and school grades as indicators of the effects of poor nutrition, it must be said that many of the investigators were forced into using such measures not because of poor science or lazy thinking, but rather because of (a) the "economicalization" of the problem of malnutrition *and* (b) the paucity of alternative measures that can predict a child's future contribution to society. Many of the large-scale intervention studies, including the Guatemalan study in which Barrett played a part, were sponsored by organizations that were concerned not merely with good science, but also with demonstrating the potential economic benefit of supplemental feeding programmes to the countries that supported them. If a supplemental feeding programme could be shown to increase some behavioural indicator of the potential earning capacity of a child, then "selling" the idea of feeding hungry children would be easy when based on a good "return" for the "investment".

But what kind of indicator can be used to predict the economic potential of a child? Developmental psychologists tend not to think in such terms, but economists and government policy makers do. They know that no perfect indicators of potential earning power exist, but they also know that IQ and school grades are, at least, correlated statistically with adult earning capacity. From such logic comes the need to demonstrate the effects of supplemental feeding progammes in terms of measures that the economist and policy makers can interpret.

The preceding argument was not intended to defend the use of insensitive indicators of the effects of poor nutrition, but rather to point out a major limitation of approaches advocated by Barrett. Although we applaud his use of "Naturalistic Intervention" as a sensitive tool for studying the effects of subtle biological and psychological variables on human behaviour, merely finding differences in behaviour between food-supplemented children and their controls is not sufficient to conclude that the children actually benefited from the supplementation programme. The danger of using such labels as "happy affect", "anxious behaviour", "social involvement", etc. to describe measurement parameters is that we invariably leap from the labels to a description of some fundamental attributes of the child. Despite Barrett's contention that: "The rating represents an assessment of the person's enduring behavioural characteristic or traits, one which presumably transcends the specifics of time and place", additional data are required before such as extrapolation is justified. It is very important to know whether children who have high ratings of "Poor frustration tolerance" are described by their peers, their teachers, their parents, etc., as having such a characteristic. Such a test would be a more valid measure of whether we are measuring "what we are trying to measure" than the method of intercorrelating response measures, as suggested by Bennett, and would be more meaningful when arguing with economists and policy makers about the effectiveness of food supplementation programmes.

Not only is it essential to validate our constructs with "real world" indicators of reality, but we must also return to the very difficult task of responding to the charge given to the earlier researchers: find an indicator in children of their potential contribution as adults. Such a challenge to the developmentalist is fraught with philosophical, theological, and political biases, but we cannot, and should not, escape from meeting it. Barrett has given us important insight into the methodologies that are sufficiently sensitive to detect the subtle effects of nutrition on behaviour, but we cannot stop there. Large-scale prospective studies, similar to the kinds described by Sinisterra, must be undertaken using the measurement techniques so adequately described by Barrett in which children must be studied for twenty-five or thirty years. The economists and policy makers must be made to articulate clearly what their critical outcome measures are, and the experimentalists must develop the methodology to measure it. Only through the execution of such a prolonged, laborious, and expensive study, will we ever learn what role is played by early dietary and other environmental variables towards determining the contribution of an individual to his/her society.

Sally Grantham-McGregor: (In response to questions from McGregor, Barrett made the following observations.)

D. E. Barrett: McGregor is correct in pointing out that the types of behaviour measures used as outcome variables in our Guatemala research are not appropriate at all age levels. We developed these measures for use with the age range of approximately 5–10 years.

It takes a very long time to develop the types of behaviour measures described in my paper. We spent about a year developing and refining the peer interaction and structural situation measures used in our study. With regard to observer training I have estimated (1) that the time necessary for training observers to use the time-sampling procedures for studying peer interaction, after the measures had been developed and refined, was 75–100 hours over a 10–12 week period.

I agree that it would be useful to have more information on the construct validity of the structural situation measures. I believe my analyses are a first step in determining the extent to which the instruments measure what they were intended to measure. Certainly, knowing the extent to which these measures are predictive of later competence would provide further support for construct validity.

McGregor is correct in her implication that several of the measures retained in the study were of only modest reliability. I included such a measure when I felt that there was a strong theoretical rationale for investigating the effects of undernutrition on that behavioural variable. I did so recognizing that I would be doing so with the relatively high risk of making a type II error (i.e. failing to identify a "true" association between variables).

For the structural situation "novel environment" there was a degree of operational dependence between outcome measures. Thus, as McGregor points out, correlations between variables within that situation might have been expected. However, the "operational dependence" does not fully explain the very high correlations between variables. For example, consider the variables "number of materials explored" and "level of exploration". One might assume that in an exploration situation, the more materials a child played with, the less time he could spend with them, and thus that the correlation would be negative. In fact, for both boys and girls it was highly positive. Boys and girls who touched many toys also played with them for longer periods. My interpretation: both variables indicate something about the child's "exploratory behaviour" (i.e., considered as a trait or characteristic). For the "competitive game structured situation", there was not operational dependence between measures. For the Impulse Control Game the variable "anticipated response" was not operationally independent of the other variables in the situation.

Across situations there was *no operational dependence between measures.* Thus, for these analyses, there was no *a priori* reason to believe that variables would be correlated, unless there was a true association between them (i.e., one not arising solely as a result of the measuring procedures used).

1. Barrett, D. E. (1982). An approach to the conceptualization and assessment of social–emotional functioning in studying nutrition–behaviour relationships. *Am. J. Clin. Nutr.* **35**, 1222–1227.

Field Studies in Early Nutrition and Later Achievement

SALLY GRANTHAM-McGREGOR

Tropical Metabolism Research Unit,
University of the West Indies, Kingston, Jamaica

This workshop focusses on early nutrition and later achievement. The term "early nutrition" includes an enormous range of conditions including overnutrition. For the purposes of this paper I will concentrate mainly on what is usually called "protein–energy malnutrition".

Protein–Energy Malnutrition

Originally protein–energy malnutrition was called protein malnutrition (1). This was then changed to protein–calorie malnutrition then protein–energy malnutrition as the importance of energy deficiency was realized. This is still not a particularly good term because it infers deficiencies of only protein and energy occurring together. However, many other types of deficiencies may occur. Figure 1, taken from Golden and Golden (2), shows some of them. There are probably more to be identified. Protein–energy malnutrition is therefore a global term referring to different conditions caused by nutrient deficiencies of varying type, degree and duration, complicated by varying amounts of infections. All of which may be inflicted at different stages of

Early Nutrition and Later Achievement
ISBN: 0-12-218855-1

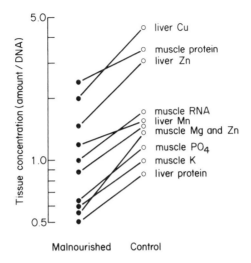

Fig. 1. Tissue concentration of protein RNA and metals in malnourished and control children. From Golden and Golden (2).

the child's development. The presently used classifications of malnutrition may be more of a hindrance than a help because they are based solely on anthropometric measurements and the presence or absence of oedema (3–5). Grouping children into a limited number of broad categories obscures the often gross metablolic heterogenicity within the groups.

The recent demonstration, in a double blind randomly controlled study, that iron supplementation affects school achievement in iron-deficient children (6), is an important finding. If one extrapolates from this, it is probable that there are other nutrient deficiencies which occur with malnutrition and affect function, but not growth.

Mechanism

The mechanism of how malnutrition may affect mental development is not established. There are several hypotheses.

(1) Permanent, anatomical and biochemical changes to the brain which affect function.

(2) Reduced exploration and activity levels of the child which lead to poor development.

(3) Reduced activity in the child subsequently produces reciprocal unresponsiveness in the child's caretakers, which in turn has a detrimental effect on the child's development.

These hypotheses are not mutually exclusive, they may occur singly or together and interact with one another: furthermore any of the above may be modified by the quality of the environment. The duration, severity of insult and age of child at the time of insult may also modify the effects.

Smart and Bedi in accompanying chapters discuss the possible changes to the brain, and maternal–child interaction has been discussed elsewhere (7,8).

Reduced activity has been reported in several studies of undernourished children (7). It is unlikely that reduced activity for a short time would have a lasting effect on a child's mental development. If this is correct, it follows that duration would be a particularly critical variable. Currently our best indicator of duration of malnutrition is attained height compared with the expected height-for-age. However, this is far from satisfactory. Not only are there many other factors affecting height apart from nutrition, but an inadequate supply of nutrients may affect height and activity differently, depending on the situation. Torun and Viteri (9) showed in children, that when energy intake was reduced in stages there was a level of intake at which normal growth continued and yet activity was reduced (Fig. 2). This was a small sample; however, if replicated, it suggests that it would be possible for energy intakes to be at levels at which activity is reduced and yet there is no concurrent reduction in linear growth. Height-for-age would therefore give an underestimation of duration of reduced activity.

Conversely, it may be possible to have situations where linear growth is restricted but activity levels are not. Several different nutrients affect linear growth, and any one of them may be limiting. When the limiting factor does not affect activity, it could result in normal activity levels in the presence

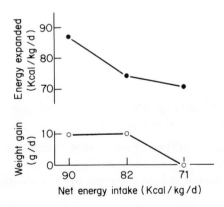

Fig. 2. Energy expenditure and weight gain of children fed 1·73 g/kg of corn and bean proteins (58:42) with changes in energy intake at 40-day intervals. From Torun and Viteri (9).

of restricted growth. This was possibly the situation in a study in Papua, New Guinea (10) when severely stunted children who were on habitually low protein diets, were given different nutritional supplements. Those given a high calorie supplement failed to catch up in height but increased in skin-fold thickness (Fig. 3). Although no measures of function were reported, it is possible that their activity levels would have increased due to the increased supply of energy, in spite of no concurrent increase in linear growth, presumably due to continued protein deficiency.

Attained height-for-age is therefore a very crude indicator of duration of reduced activity and we need a better one.

The present classification of "severe malnutrition" which combines marasmus and kwashiorkor further confuses attempts to find an association between poor mental development and malnutrition. Oedema is the *sine qua non*

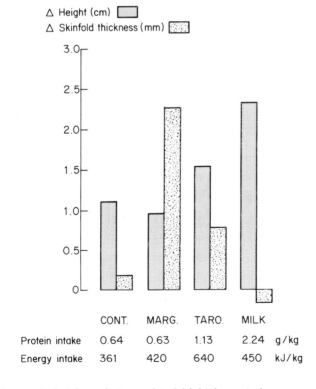

	CONT.	MARG.	TARO.	MILK	
Protein intake	0.64	0.63	1.13	2.24	g/kg
Energy intake	361	420	640	450	kJ/kg

Fig. 3. Changes in height and triceps skin-fold thickness in four groups of children from Papua, New Guinea, over a 13 week period. The groups received no supplement (cont), 30 g margarine (marg.) increased staple diet (taro) and skim milk powder per day. From data of Malcolm (10); figure from Golden and Golden (2).

of kwashiorkor (4), but oedema rarely persists for more than a few weeks. If the presence of oedema *per se* is linked to poor mental development the possible mechanisms are difficult to discern.

Most studies comparing the later development of children who have recovered from severe malnutrition, with that of control groups, have found the malnourished children have significantly poorer function (11). Two of the few exceptions involve South African children who survived kwashiorkor. Evans and colleagues (12) found that survivors of kwashiorkor had similar IQs and school achievement levels to a control group of siblings. Bartel and colleagues (13) found in another group of survivors of kwashiorkor that they had similar scores on tests of motor development, grip strength, finger tapping and motor speed to those of two control groups of siblings and yard mates. Hoorweg and Stanfield in a study of survivors of severe PEM in Uganda (14) failed to find an association between signs of kwashiorkor and levels of mental development several years later, although they did find an association with signs of marasmus. Similarly in Jamaica (15), we studied children who were in hospital with severe malnutrition and failed to find an association between the presence of oedema and developmental levels one month after they left hospital. However, there was an association with height deficit.

Although kwashiorkor is associated with gross behavioural abnormalities in the acute stage these disappear on recovery. Considering the above, I would like to hypothesize that any long-term effects of kwashiorkor on mental development are linked to the underlying chronic undernutrition rather than to the transient episode of oedema. One way of testing this hypothesis would be to compare the development of chronically undernourished children without a history of oedema, with other children who had a similar degree of undernutrition at the same age but also had an episode of oedema.

In spite of all the above reservations, we have not devised a better way of classifying malnutrition than by anthropometric criteria. Until our technology improves it is necessary to use standard classifications in order to facilitate comparisons between populations and between research findings. In this chapter I will use the Wellcome Classification terminology (4). In future studies it would be better to use stunting as a measure of chronic undernutrition and wasting as a measure of recent nutritional experiences (5) and not include kwashiorkor with severe malnutrition, but, look at it separately.

Despite the reservations of uncomplicated kwashiorkor an association between poor mental development and childhood protein--energy malnutrition has been repeatedly demonstrated over the last 30 or more years. However, there remains doubt as to whether and in what circumstances this relationship is causal.

Studies suffer from many difficulties apart from those of diagnosing malnutrition. Pollitt and Thomson (11) have discussed the problems of validity and reliability when measuring cognitive functioning in countries where there are no indigenous tests. Perhaps the greatest problem facing investigators however is that malnutrition in developing countries is inevitably associated with a host of sociocultural disadvantages which themselves have a detrimental effect on mental development. The recent history of research in this area has largely involved attempts at separating these effects from those of malnutrition.

There are several reviews of studies in the field (11,16) and it would be redundant to further review each one in detail. Instead, I will discuss the issues emerging from these studies, attempting to give the perspective of someone who has worked with malnourished children for many years.

Observational Studies

By far the greatest number of studies of children who have suffered severe malnutrition have been retrospective case-control observational ones. Survivors of severe malnutrition have been identified and investigated several years after recovery (e.g. 14,17,18). A further group of studies have followed up children from the time they suffered from one acute episode (e.g. 19,20), usually comparing them with a control group. After the realization that poor social backgrounds were major confounding variables, heroic steps have been taken to match for possible differences in backgrounds. Investigators have used siblings or carefully matched subjects as controls, or measured sociocultural variables and controlled for them statistically. However, none of the approaches have been entirely satisfactory (21).

Comparing survivors with siblings merely reduces the effects of malnutrition because the siblings themselves were almost certainly undernourished in early childhood. Usually there are also differences in birth order and sometimes sex and age range. To identify and measure all social background factors which may affect development is impossible, although these studies have the advantage of highlighting the important contribution of social background to mental development (21).

A further problem in identifying children several years after the episode, is that we have little idea of what happened in the interim and probably no measure of development immediately following the acute episode. It is therefore not safe to infer that children who have higher IQs at follow-up have "caught up", as they may never have had low levels of development in the first place. There is a similar problem with control children; only few studies have records of their nutritional status in early childhood (18) and they may well have been undernourished themselves. There is the further danger that children lost to follow-up are not representative and therefore bias the resulting sample, probably in favour of better performance.

Considering the large number of reported studies, and their inherent difficulties, it may be concluded that further observational studies of this kind are unlikely to help us identify a causal relationship between severe malnutrition and mental development and should be discouraged. The one consistent finding from retrospective studies is that children suffering from marasmus in early childhood have poorer levels of mental development than matched peers or siblings many years later, if they return to deprived environments (11).

Studies which begin with children already suffering from malnutrition cannot tell us whether the children were normal before the episode. Prospective studies beginning before malnutrition develops offer many advantages over retrospective ones; however they are difficult to carry out, not only for logistical but also for ethical reasons. It is not possible to make a purely observational study of children becoming malnourished so that children who develop malnutrition do so in spite of the vigorous attempts of the investigators to prevent it. This may bias the sample to an unacceptable degree. However, in the only reported prospective study beginning before the onset of malnutrition, Cravioto and Delicardie (22) demonstrated in a Mexican village that children who became severely malnourished had similar levels of psychomotor development to the other village children, prior to the onset of malnutrition.

Studies in Developed Countries

Observational studies of children who suffer malnutrition secondary to clinical disease in developed countries are one way of separating poor nutrition from poor social backgrounds. Several of these studies have shown that the children have very little or no deficit in mental functioning several years later (23). However, at least one showed that children who were tested at a younger age had poorer levels of mental development than their matched controls, but children tested at an older age did not. It would be interesting to know whether or not the children suffered a temporary set back in development following the episode of illness and then recovered.

It is probable that the duration of malnutrition in these children was not as long as it was in children studied in underdeveloped countries. In addition, on recovery the children would have returned to good nutrition, in stark contrast to survivors of severe malnutrition in poor countries who usually return to chronically inadequate diets.

More importantly, the environmental context of malnutrition may be critical. It has been shown in rats that increased stimulation reduces the detrimental effects of food deprivation on behaviour (24,25), so that these children may have been protected from possible harmful effects of malnutrition by an enrichment environment, or have compensated for them.

Intervention Studies

Intervention studies which use experimental or quasi-experimental designs allow us to come closer to inferring cause. They appear to be a definite step forward from observational studies, both in terms of research design and in terms of providing possible guidelines for future service programmes.

I intend to focus on these studies for the rest of this paper. Most comprise studies of nutritional supplementation given to populations exposed to chronic undernutrition starting either from pregnancy or birth, somewhat fewer have looked at the effects of supplementation given to children who have already become undernourished or severely malnourished. These studies attempt to isolate the effects of nutrition from those of social background. A few have looked at the effects of enriching the social environment of undernourished children and only one has attempted to look for possible interaction between social and nutritional factors. First I will briefly mention their main findings then discuss the issues arising from them. Tables 1 and 2 list the studies in developing countries.

Populations Exposed to Malnutrition

Pregnancy only

We could find no studies from developing countries of supplementation restricted to pregnancy and measuring subsequent psychomotor development. In New York (16), supplementation of pregnant high-risk women had no effect on their children's psychomotor development at 1 year of age. In Montreal, Canada (26) supplementation of pregnant mothers showed no benefit to their children's school achievement.

Pregnancy and lactation

In a double-blind, randomly assigned study in Taiwan (27), supplementation to mothers in pregnancy and lactation was found to have a small but significant benefit on children's scores on the motor scale of the Bayley Test at 8 months of age, but not on the mental scale.

Table 1. Intervened studies in children exposed to undernutrition in developing countries.

Location	Sample selection	Groups	Results
Bogota, Colombia (28,29,30, 56,61)	433 high-risk families randomly assigned to six groups. Treatment lasted until child was 3 years old	(1) Early supplement (2) Late supplement (3) Continual supplement (4) Stimulation (5) Stimulation and supplement (6) No treatment	Supplement gave small benefits to Griffiths DQ. Moderate increase in activity at 4 months. Early supplement not different from late. Stimulation gave small benefit to language development
Guatemala (31,32,53,54)	Self-selected from 4 villages 1083 children supplement given in pregnancy, lactation and up to 7 years	High supplementation compared with low supplementation	Small association between level of supplement and cognitive functioning on INCAP preschool battery
Taiwan (27)	255 pregnant, high-risk, mothers, randomly assigned to groups. Children not treated	(1) Mothers received a placebo drink (2) Supplemented throughout pregnancy and lactation	Small benefit in motor scale of Bayley
Mexico (33)	40 pregnant women in one village assigned to 2 groups separated by time of birth. Supplementation throughout pregnancy and lactation and children for at least 3 years.	(1) Children born in 1 year supplemented. (2) Children born 1–2 years previously, not supplemented	Marked DQ benefit on Gesel, marked increase in activity
South Africa (34)	14 sibling pairs assigned to 2 groups. Child received supplement from 2 to 28 months	(1) Older siblings received no treatment (2) Younger siblings supplemented	Marked IQ benefit on South African Intelligence Scale, etc.
Louisiana (35)	21 sibling pairs in low-income families received supplement	(1) Older siblings supplemented after 1 year for 30 months (2) Younger sibling supplemented from pregnancy to 56 months	Marked IQ benefit on WISC and other tests to younger siblings.

Table 2. Intervention studies of nutritional supplementation in undernourished or severely malnourished children.

Location	Sample selection	Samples	Impact on development
Cali, Colombia (37)	1st pilot: undernourished children, number, age, group assignment not given, treatment 4 months 2nd pilot: undernourished and adequately nourished children, number, age not given. Treatment 5 months	(1) Cognitive stimulation (2) Physical stimulation (3) Nut. supplement (4) No treatment (1–3) Control groups (4 & 5) Stimulation + supplement (6) Supplementation alone	(1 & 2) Marked benefit to tests of general cognitive ability. (3) No benefit (4 & 5) Marked benefits to cognitive functioning. (6) Supplement increased activity level only
Cali, Colombia (37)	301 3-year-old children living in two poor urban areas, lowest weight and height. Randomly assigned to seven groups	Four groups each receiving different periods of stimulation and supplementation, 3 groups each receiving different periods of supplementation	Stimulation with supplementation had marked benefit to WISC IQ and school achievement tests, increasing with duration. Supplementation alone, no benefit
Bogota Colombia (36)	186 undernourished and 192 adequately nourished sibling pairs, aged 6 to 60 months. Group assignment not given. Treatment for 1 year	(1) Well nourished supplemented (2) Well nourished unsupplemented (3) Undernourished supplemented (4) Undernourished unsupplemented	Supplement made small benefits to Griffiths DQ in undernourished only
Narangwal, India (39)	Villages assigned to different combinations of health care and supplementation, children below cutoff points given supplementation. Total of 479 randomly selected from each village	(1) Health care (2) Suppl. and health care (3) Suppl. alone (4) Nothing	(2) Small benefit to fine and gross motor development in locally designed test. No other significant benefits
Chile (40)	14 recovered severely malnourished children given supplement	No controls	Very low IQs between 3 and 6 years

Pregnancy and early childhood

Two large studies of nutritional supplementation during pregnancy and early childhood were carried out in Latin America.

Bogota, Colombia. In Bogota (28) pregnant mothers who already had undernourished children were randomly assigned to groups: one group received nutritional supplementation in pregnancy and through the first three years of the infant's life: one group received increased stimulation for the first three years: another group received both treatments; and a fourth group received no treatment. At 18 months of age (29) supplementation had a significant benefit on all subscales of the Griffiths Test except language, but by 36 months (28) language also showed a benefit. In contrast, stimulation had a benefit on language and personal social subscales at 18 months and only on the language subscale at 36 months. The stimulation effects decreased with age. A significant interaction between supplementation and stimulation was reported in two subscales at 18 months but not at 36 months. All benefits both from supplementation and stimulation were small. There were two additional groups; one received supplementation in pregnancy and throughout the first six months of the infant's life, and this group was not different from the other which received supplementation from 6 to 36 months. Stimulation affected caretaker's responsiveness and interaction with the child at both 4 and 8 months of age (30), whereas supplementation affected the child's positive activity level, especially in stimulated children at 4 months. There were no main effects of supplementation at 8 months.

Guatemala. In Guatemala (31) 4 villages participated in a nutritional supplementation project. Two villages received a high protein drink (atole) and two a low calorie drink (fresco) from a central feeding station. Supplement was available on a self-selection basis. There was a significant association between the amount of supplement eaten and cognitive functioning. Supplement was reported to favour the more motoric and manipulative skills rather than linguistic and cognitive ones up to 3 years of age (32). However, after 3 years of age this was not the case and language development showed the greatest benefit, however, all effects were small and a full analysis has not yet been reported.

Mexico. In a much smaller study in a Mexican village, Chavez and Martinez (33) supplemented 20 mothers and children throughout pregnancy and early childhood (it is not clear for how long). The children were compared with another group of unsupplemented children born one year previously in the same village. The supplemented group showed a remarkable increase in activity levels and exploration. The mothers in turn showed more responsive-ness to their supplemented children, and this was interpreted as the more active exploring child invoking more stimulating behaviour in the mother. The supplemented children attained markedly higher scores on the Gesel Schedules between 6 and 60 months of age, than the unsupplemented ones.

Two additional studies involving small groups of siblings had unusually large benefits in IQ scores.

South Africa. In South Africa (34) 14 children born into families which already had had a child who suffered from kwashiorkor, were supplemented from 2 months to 28 months of age. Their mean IQs at 9 years of age were 10 points higher than their non-supplementated sibling who preceded them but did not have kwashiorkor.

Louisiana, USA. In the USA (35) 21 children who had received supplementation from pregnancy for an average of 56 months were compared with their older siblings who had received supplement only after one year of age for an average of 31 months. At 6 and 8 years, respectively, there was a difference of 13 IQ points on the WISC.

Nutritional Supplementation with Malnourished Children

Bogota, Colombia. In Bogota (36) pairs of undernourished and adequately nourished siblings were assigned to two treatment groups: one group received nutritional supplementation for 1 year, and the other group received no treatment. Supplementation produced a small benefit to the developmental quotients on the Griffiths Test in undernourished children only, although both supplemented groups improved in weight. The children ranged in age from 4 to 66 months and no report could be found of a breakdown by age, or by subscale of the Griffiths Test.

Cali, Colombia. Two pilot studies (37) preceded the large study described below. These are of great interest but unfortunately no details were reported. The first lasted four months and groups of undernourished children were exposed to different types of interventions: cognitive stimulation, physical stimulation, food and health care, and nothing. All treatments were given at a local centre. The children receiving food and health care only showed no benefit at all to their development. However, the cognitive stimulation group showed marked benefits; the physical stimulation group also showed improvement, but slightly less so.

A second study which lasted five months also tested different intervention strategies using both undernourished and adequately nourished but deprived children. Cognitive stimulation produced benefits to both types of children, but the group which received food and health alone, this time at home, showed no improvements at tests of reading or cognitive function. They were however reported to have increased activity levels, although details are not given.

Cali, Colombia. Following the above study, a large study was conducted (38) in which nutritional supplementation with or without an early childhood educational component, was given to poor and chronically undernourished 3-year-old children.

Nutritional supplementation alone had no effect on their scores on tests of cognitive function. However, in combination with the educational component, the children showed impressive improvements which were proportional to the duration of the programme. They did not separate stimulation alone from stimulation plus food, so it is not possible to discern if nutritional supplementation improved the benefits of stimulation or not.

Narangwal, India. A "comprehensive" nutrition and health care project in Narangwal, India (39), offered different combinations of nutritional supplementation and health care to different villages. Where supplementation was offered, it was only given to children whose nutritional status was below certain cut-off points. Evaluation of a random group of children from each village indicated that children in the village which was given supplementation and health care had higher scores on psychomotor testing in gross and fine motor development than did those in the control village. However, no attempt was made to link supplement or dietary intake to development.

Chile. The only report I could find on the effects of long-term supplementation on the mental development in children recovering from severe malnutrition comes from Chile (40). Monckeberg studied 14 children for several years after recovering from the acute stage of protein–energy malnutrition. He gave all the young children in the family 20 litres of milk each a month. There were neither control groups nor records of intakes, however, the children's IQs were very low between 3 and 6 years. Their weights were reported as "normal" but their heights "low"; the actual data was not presented.

Psychosocial Stimulation and Severely Malnourished Children

Short-term

These studies have been reviewed in more detail elsewhere (41). All of them concerned stimulation while children were recovering from severe malnutrition in hospital (42–46). Only three of these had control groups (42–44) and report short-term improvements in developmental quotients (DQ). However, in two of the studies (47,48) benefits gained were lost 1 year later. No long-term report of the third study could be found (44).

Long-term

The only reported programme of long-term psychosocial stimulation with severely malnourished children is one we have just completed in Jamaica (49–51). The intervention was designed to be integrated into the existing primary health care services. It comprised an hour's play a day while the children were in hospital, followed by home visiting for 1 hour a week for 2 years, then every 2 weeks for a further year. Community health aides (paraprofessionals employed by the Jamaican government) conducted the visits. At the visits, they demonstrated the use of home-made toys to the mothers, in an attempt to make them more effective teachers of their children. The mothers were encouraged to play with their children between the visits.

The intervened malnourished group ($n = 21$) was compared with two other groups who were patients in the same hospital one year previously, and had received standard medical care only. These comprised a second severely malnourished group ($n = 18$) and an adequately nourished one ($n = 21$).

On admission to hospital both malnourished groups were seriously behind the adequately nourished group on developmental testing. The non-intervened malnourished group remained behind the adequately nourished children for the following 6 years showing little sign of catching up. The intervened malnourished children showed improvement in developmental levels and were significantly ahead of the non-intervened malnourished group by the time they left hospital. They continued to improve and twelve months later their DQs were similar to those of the adequately nourished group. They maintained this position for a second year but showed a slight decline in the third year of intervention. In the three years following intervention they showed a gradual decline, but remained ahead of the non-intervened malnourished group. The test scores standardized at each test point are shown in Fig. 4.

Language development responded the fastest to stimulation, and locomotor development was the one area of development in which they did not catch up to the well-nourished group. Both malnourished groups remained stunted with small head circumferences compared with the adequately nourished group, even up to six years after leaving hospital. The intervention did not include nutritional supplementation.

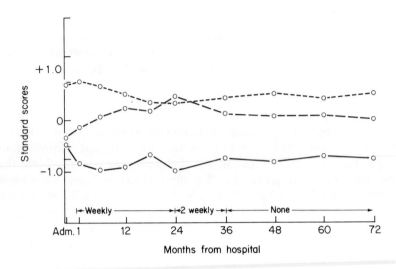

Fig. 4. Developmental and intelligence quotients transformed to standard scores for each test session from admission to hospital to 72 months following discharge for three groups: adequately nourished (dotted line); non-intervened malnourished (solid line); and intervened malnourished (broken line). From Grantham-McGregor *et al.* (51).

Issues Arising from Intervention Studies

There are many issues arising from the above studies, and I will discuss the main ones under the following headings: study design; measurements: subjects; treatment: mechanism; and outcomes.

Study Design

Random assignment to groups is essential if one is to infer cause. However, the only studies to have random assignment were those in New York (16), Taiwan (27), Cali, Colombia (38) and Bogota (28). In some studies the precise method of assignment is not clear (36,37,42). There are many reasons for the lack of randomization: it is not always possible to deliver different treatments to children living in a crowded neighbourhood, where families know each other; it has even been found to be difficult to deliver different levels of stimulation to children in the same hospital (43).

In order to solve this problem investigators have chosen different groups from different neighbourhoods, villages (31,39) or hospitals (44). This leads to mismatching because inevitably differences emerge after commencement of the study which were not originally considered. For example, in the

Guatemalan study, villages differed on reasons why children attended school. We have also had this experience in Jamaica, where differences emerged in the quality of neighbourhood schools.

Studies with no controls at all are not possible to interpret (40,45,46) neither are ones where the treatment delivered to individual subjects is not reported (39).

Having controls separated in time is another common fault (26,34,35,49). In this case, it is not possible to be sure that events outside the study are not responsible for the outcome. In the sibling studies referred to above (34,35), not only were the children separated in time, but there was an age difference between the groups at the time of IQ testing, as well as a birth order difference.

Studies in which supplement was taken on a self-selection basis, and then groups with high and low levels of ingestion compared (31), present serious problems. The supplemented children may represent a different population. For example, the group with highest intakes may have the greatest need or have the most sensible mothers. The act of consuming the supplement, where it is dispensed at a central feeding station, may also be very stimulating, and benefit the child independently of the nutrient effect.

The extra attention focussed on supplemented children might also have an "inadvertent" benefit on their behaviour. This is especially so where only one subject in the family is fed, and may partly explain the marked improvement found in the Mexican study (33). Some studies overcame this by providing a placebo (27,16). Where the subjects are undernourished children, providing them with non-nutritious food is a difficult ethical decision, especially if it is dispensed by health personnel. Feeding the whole family was attempted in the Bogota study (28), and this may lessen the individual attention focussed on the child. However, when interpreting findings it must be remembered that any change in the children's level of development may have a different aetiology. A better diet may change the behaviour of other family members who might then interact differently with the children. In the Mexican study (33) mothers were fed through lactation until the next pregnancy. In this study marked changes in the mother's behaviour have been recorded, and these have generally been attributed to changes in the child's behaviour. We have generally ignored the possible effect of improvements in the mother's diet on her behaviour.

The question of the effects of improved diets to the whole family is however an important and socially relevant one.

Measurement

I will not go into the problems of using culturally inappropriate tests which have been discussed elsewhere (11). Nor will I address the problem of measuring different outcome variables such as behaviour, as this is being discussed by Brožek in this workshop. However, the difficulty of testing the mental development of large numbers of children in the field cannot be overemphasized.

Deprived children in the first 4 years of life are particularly shy and withdrawn in the testing situation. Skilled testers are needed who should have at least a college education. Several studies report a "tester effect". All testers should be spread equally across groups and "tester" should be accounted for in the analysis. In longitudinal studies it is difficult to keep the same testers over time. Where groups are separated by time this may present serious problems.

As Rush (16) pointed out, the fluctuation in test scores in the Bogota study (28) are difficult to explain, even taking into account that the Griffiths Test was not developed in Colombia. The changing scores might, at least partly, reflect the logistics of large-scale testing over long periods of time.

Subjects

Different types of subjects may respond differently to the same treatment, and this may explain some inconsistencies in findings. In supplementation studies the subject's initial nutritional status and habitual dietary intake affects their growth response. The more malnourished the children are, the more likely they are to respond in growth (52). Also subjects with adequate habitual diets are unlikely to respond (53). Only one study has addressed the effect of the subject's initial nutritional status on their response in development (36). In this study undernourished children showed improvements in development with supplementation, whereas adequately nourished ones did not.

Failure to find improved development in children born to mothers who were supplemented in developed countries (16,26) may be explained by their habitual diets being adequate, or at least not lacking in the constituents of the supplement.

It is not clear what influence the subject's age has on their response. Maximum response to nutritional supplementation in weight and height was reported in the first three years of life (54) however, good growth response has been reported after three years (36,55). It was originally thought that the last trimester of pregnancy and first 6 months of life were critical in the relationship between undernutrition and development. The Bogota (28) and Guatemalan study (31) have not substantiated this. However, all children in these studies were predominantly breastfed so that the difference in nutritional status between control and supplemented groups would have been very little in the first few months of life (54,56). Dietary intakes were not measured in either study in the first year. It may be that, where lactation does not fail, malnutrition in the first 3 months is highly unlikely to occur, even in poor communities. In observational studies of survivors of severe malnutrition, the children below 6 months have not been shown to be more vulnerable than older children (14).

The striking finding of absolutely no effect of supplementation on tests of cognitive function of undernourished 3-year-old children in two studies in Cali, Colombia (37,38), may be associated with the somewhat older age of the children. The authors of longitudinal studies have not fully analysed their results by age (31).

The effect of stimulation may also vary by subject's age. It is well known that social background variables explain more of the variance in mental development as the child gets older. There is some evidence that stimulation is less effective in the first year of life than in older children (57).

Whether the nutritional status of the children affects the response of the children to stimulation is unknown. Only one pilot study in Cali, Colombia (37) has looked at this directly, and unfortunately that was poorly documented. Cognitive stimulation was provided to two groups of deprived children, an undernourished group and an adequately nourished one. Both groups improved to a marked extent but not to the same degree in different aspects of development. However, the programme only lasted 5 months. In Jamaica, deprived but adequately nourished children, showed a marked benefit of 13 DQ points from a home visiting programme lasting 9 months (58). There is ample evidence from the USA of improvement in performance on intelligence testing (59), at least in the short term, following early childhood stimulation programmes.

Treatment

Most nutritional supplementation studies have had disappointing results in terms of growth (60). The main reason is probably that insufficient amounts of nutrients reach the target subjects either through failure to collect the food, sharing it, substituting it for the usual diets, or high morbidity rates.

In the studies reviewed most have had either no report of dietary intake (34–40) or inadequate assessments such as one isolated 24-hour dietary recall.

Careful records of supplement ingestion (31) are no substitute for total dietary intake. In fact they give a misleading impression of accuracy when substitution is not accounted for. When dietary intake data is reported, the actual increase is usually very modest compared with the amount of supplementation offered. For example, the increase in the Bogota study (61) was 840 kJ per day and the difference in intake between children taking fresco and atole in the Guatemalan study averaged 420 kJ per day (62).

The growth response in most of the reviewed studies was small, rarely amounting to more than a centimetre a year (e.g. in Bogota (56) and in Guatemala (54)). The effect of supplement on development should be seen in terms of the increase in actual intake, not the amount of supplement offered.

In those studies where neither growth nor dietary intake is reported, and there was no response in development, it is impossible to interpret the results of supplementation with any degree of certainty (35,36). It may be relevant that the Mexican study reported exceptionally good growth and also some of the largest improvements in development (33). It is also possible that the composition of the supplement may be important; for example if the habitual diet is adequate in protein but not energy, high energy supplement would be the most effective (55).

Many of the issues related to psychosocial stimulation have been discussed elsewhere (41), so I will not reiterate them here. There has been little documented attempt to standardize the quality of home visits, and this is a major problem with home programmes. Also, it is usually unclear what stimulation programmes actually comprise. The possible effects of the social and emotional support of having a friendly visitor going to the home has not been separated from the effects of direct stimulation of the child.

The evidence is reasonably conclusive that short-term stimulation has transient effects only. There were three studies of long-term stimulation. Those in Jamaica (50) and Cali (38) produced marked benefits, whereas the Bogota study (28) had very small benefits. In Bogota stimulation started from birth, in contrast to the other two studies which started with older, malnourished children.

In all three studies, the greatest gain occurred early in the study. In both Jamaica and Bogota the gains decreased with time. Both these interventions used similar strategies which comprised home visiting with maternal education. The reason for the decline is not clear; however in Jamaica we had the impression that both mothers and visitors wearied of the programme towards the end, and the number of visits was reduced in the last year. The children in the Cali study actually increased their gains with time. This was a centre-based study, and it is unlikely that professional teachers would have experienced "programme fatigue".

The poorer response to increased stimulation in Bogota than in Jamaica is probably related either to differences in the children or differences in the treatment. It is difficult to control the quality of home visits, and the smaller size of the Jamaican study would have facilitated supervision; in addition we had a locally designed curriculum and probably more play materials. However, in Bogota the visits were more frequent and the visitors better educated.

Mechanism

Where benefits to development from nutrition supplementation have been found, we have little idea as to the mechanism. Increased activity and exploration may play a part. Unfortunately few studies have measured this. The Mexico (33) and Bogota (30) studies reported increased activity levels, with a much higher increase in Mexico than in Bogota. The Mexican children also showed greater improvements in development. However, activity levels in the supplemented children did not show a marked increase until after 4 months of age, at which time a large difference in development was already apparent.

One of the pilot studies in Cali, Colombia (37) found that supplementation for five months in undernourished children increased activity levels but there was no increase in tests of cognitive functions.

There is therefore no adequate data to show that increased activity is mechanistic in producing improved levels of functioning. Indeed it is possible that increased activity in a deprived environment may be not be sufficient to produce benefits in development unless the environment is also improved.

Outcomes

Nutritional supplementation

Findings from studies of nutritional supplementation, have been inconsistent. In developed countries supplementation in pregnancy produced no benefits in psychomotor development (16). In nutritionally deprived populations, supplementation in pregnancy and lactation produced very small benefits (27); when extended to early childhood small (28,31) or marked (33–35) benefits were found.

In undernourished children either no (37,38) or very small effects were found (36). Where benefits were found there was a tendency to favour motor development (27,29,32) in the first two years of life.

Psychosocial stimulation

Psychosocial stimulation has produced marked benefits in undernourished or severely malnourished children exposed to long-term treatments (38,50). Only one study (28) began from birth and this has very small benefits. There is a suggestion that language development responds the most (28) or the quickest (49) to stimulation.

Nutritional supplementation and stimulation interaction

It is not possible from published data to determine whether there is an interaction between supplementation and stimulation. Only the Bogota study (28) had an appropriate study design to look for this, and that study had unusually poor results from stimulation and wide variation in scores between tests. They did, however, show a small interaction effect at 18 months (29).

Long-term effects

I have only discussed concurrent or short-term effects of interventions so far. However, several studies have now reported follow-up findings. In the Bogota study (63) 7-year-old children who had received nutritional supplementation performed better at school readiness tests. The only benefit from stimulation was that the children enrolled in school earlier. There was a significant effect of both supplementation and stimulation on the number of children repeating grades. Both supplementation and stimulation, alone or combined, resulted in heavier and taller children.

Stimulated children in the Cali study (64) made greater progress through the first three grades in school and had higher IQ scores at 9 years than control children. Benefits remained proportional to the duration of treatment.

In Jamaica (51) intervened children had higher IQs 3 years after intervention than non-intervened malnourished children.

In Mexico (65) the supplemented children performed better in first grade and were more alert, attentive and active than non-supplemented children.

It would seem that most of the studies which have looked for long-term effects have found very small ones. Considering the large amount of effort invested in the longitudinal studies, it would seem justified to follow children, from at least some of the studies, into adulthood and look at other social and economic parameters. In the USA children who participated in early childhood interventions have been shown to have many benefits in "real life" outcomes such as less delinquency, fewer teenage pregnancies, better progress in school, and greater access to employment (66).

Conclusions

The intervention studies reviewed represent an enormous investment in time, money and toil, and we have learnt a considerable amount about the development of deprived children. In spite of this, inconsistent findings, flaws in study design and differences in treatments and subjects, preclude making firm conclusions.

It is apparent that both nutritional supplementation and stimulation affects development in children in some circumstances. But in which subjects, with which type of treatment and to what extent, and whether there is an interaction between treatments, remains uncertain. Of all the studies reviewed, only the Bogota (24) and Cali (34) ones attempted to look at the effects of improving both the nutritional status and psychosocial environment. This would seem by far the most sensible approach if we are concerned with malnutrition as it occurs in the "real world". The Bogota study is unique in attempting to assess the effects of both these interventions, alone and combined.

It is clear that programmes of nutritional supplementation alone will not solve the problems of poor development in chronically undernourished deprived children to any great extent. However, we must be careful not to conclude that undernutrition is unimportant to development, in the light of the inadequate nature of data currently available.

References

1. WHO (1953). World Health Organization Technical Report Series. No. 72. Geneva.
2. Golden, M. H. and Golden, B. E. (1985) Trace elements in malnutrition. In "Spurenelemente" (E. Gladrke, G. Heiman, I. Lombeck and I. Eckert, eds) pp. 47–57. Georg Thieme Verlag, Stuttgart and New York.
3. Gomez, F. R., Galvan, R., Cravioto, J. and Frenk, S. (1954). Malnutrition in infancy and childhood with special reference to kwashiorkor. *Adv. Pediat.* 7, 131–169.
4. Editorial (1970) Classification of infantile malnutrition. *Lancet* ii, 302.
5. Waterlow, J. C. and Rutishauser, H. E. (1974). Malnutrition in man. *In* "Early Malnutrition and Mental Development" (J. Cravioto, L. Hambreus and B. Vahlquist, eds). pp. 13–25. Almquist and Witsel, Uppsala.
6. Soemantri, A. G., Pollitt, E. and Kim, I. (1985). Iron deficiency anaemia and educational achievement. *Am. J. Clin. Nutr.* 42, 1221–1228.
7. Grantham-McGregor, S. M. (1984). Social background of childhood malnutrition. *In* "Malnutrition and Behavior: Critical Assessment of Key Issues," (J. Brožek and B. Schürch, eds) pp. 358–375. Nestlé Foundation, Lausanne, Switzerland.
8. Galler, J. R., Ricciuti, H. N., Crawford, M. A. and Kucharski, L. T. (1984). The role of the mother–infant interaction in nutritional disorders. *In* "Human Nutrition: A Comprehensive Treatise" (J. R. Galler, ed.) pp. 269–300. Plenum Press, New York.
9. Torun, B. and Viteri, F. E. (1981). Energy requirements of preschool children and effects of varying energy intakes on protein metabolism. *In* "Protein–energy Requirements of Developing Countries; Evaluation of New Data," (B. Torun, V. R. Young and W. M. Rand, eds) pp. 229–247. United Nations Uni. Food Nutri. Bull. (Suppl. 5), Tokyo.

10. Malcolm, L. A. (1970). Growth retardation in a New Guinea boarding school and its response to supplementary feeding. *Brit. J. Nutr.* **24**, 297–305.
11. Pollitt, E. and Thomson, C. (1977). Protein–calorie malnutrition and behaviour. A view from psychology. *In* "Nutrition and Brain" (R. J. Wurtmann and J. J. Wurtmann, eds) Vol. 2, pp. 261–306. Raven Press, New York.
12. Evans, D. E., Moodie, A. D. and Hansen, J. D. L. (1971). Kwashiorkor and intellectual development. *S. Afr. Med. J.* **25**, 1413–1426.
13. Bartel, P. R., Griesel, R. D., Burnett, L. S., Freiman, I., Rosen, E. V. and Geefhuysen, J. (1971). Long term effects of kwashiorkor on psychomotor development. *S. Afr. Med. J.* **53**, 360–362.
14. Hoorweg, J. and Stanfield, J. P. (1976). The effects of protein energy malnutrition in early childhood and intellectual and motor abilities in later childhood and adolescence. *Dev. Med. Child Neurol.* **18**, 330–350.
15. Grantham-McGregor, S. M. (1982). The relationship between development level and different types of malnutrition in children. *Human Nutr., Clin. Nutr.* **36C**, 319–320.
16. Rush, D. (1984). The behavioural consequences of protein–energy deprivation and supplementation in early life: An epidemiological perspective. *In* "Human Nutrition: A Comprehensive Treatise" (J. Galler, ed.) pp. 119–154, Plenum Press, New York.
17. Hertzig, M. E., Birch, H. G., Richardson, S. A. and Tizard, J. (1972). Intellectual levels of school children severely malnourished during the first two years of life. *Pediat.* **49**, 814–824.
18. Galler, J., Ramsey, F., Solimano, G., Lowell, W. E. and Mason, E. (1983). The influence of early malnutrition on subsequent behavioural development 1. Degree of impairment in intellectual performance. *J. Am. Acad. Child. Psych.* **22**, 8–15.
19. Stoch, M. B., Smythe, P. M., Moodie, A. D. and Bradshaw, D. (1982). Psychological outcome and CT findings after gross undernourishment during infancy; a 20-year developmental study. *Dev. Med. Child Neurol.* **24**, 419–436.
20. Grantham-McGregor, S. M., Powell, C., Stewart, M. and Schofield, W. N. (1982). Longitudinal study of growth and development of young Jamaican children recovering from severe protein–energy malnutrition. *Dev. Med. Child Neurol.* **24**, 321–331.
21. Richardson, S. A. (1976). The relation of severe malnutrition in infancy to the intelligence of school children with differing life histories. *Pediat. Res.* **10**, 57–61.
22. Cravioto, J. and Delicardie, E. (1972). Environmental correlates of severe clinical malnutrition and language development in survivors from kwashiorkor or marasmus. *In* "Nutrition, The Nervous System and Behaviour", P.A.H.O. Scientific Publication No. 251, pp. 73–94. Washington.
23. Lloyd-Still, J. D. (1976). Clinical studies on the effects of malnutrition during infancy and subsequent physical and intellectual development. *In* "Malnutrition and Intellectual Development" (J. D. Lloyd-Still, ed.) pp. 103–140. MTP Press Ltd, Lancaster.
24. Levitsky, D. (1979). Malnutrition and the hunger to learn. *In* "Malnutrition, Environment and Behaviour" (D. A. Levitsky, ed.) pp. 161–179. Cornell University Press, Ithaca and London.
25. Fraňková, S. (1979). Behavioural consequences of early malnutrition and environmental stimuli. *In* "Malnutrition, Environment and Behaviour" (D. A. Levitsky, ed.) pp. 149–160. Cornell University Press, Ithaca and London.

26. Pencharz, P., Heller, A., Higgins, A., Strawbridge, J., Rush, D. and Pless, B. (1983). Effects of nutritional services to pregnant mothers on the school performance of treated and untreated children. *Nutr. Res.* **3**, 795–803.

27. Joos, S. K., Pollitt, E. Mueller, W. H. and Albright, D. L. (1983). The Bacon Chow Study: Maternal nutritional supplementation and infant behavioural development. *Child Dev.* **54**, 669–676.

28. Waber, D. P., Vuori-Christiansen, L., Ortiz, N., Clement, J., Christiansen, N. E., Mora, J. O., Reed, R. B. and Herrera, G. H. (1981). Nutritional supplementation, maternal education and cognitive development of infants at risk of malnutrition. *Am. J. Clin. Nutr.* **34**, 801–813.

29. Mora, J. O., Clement, J., Christiansen, N., Ortiz, N. Vuori, L. and Wagner, M. (1979). Nutritional supplementation early stimulation and child development. *In* "Behavioural Effects of Energy and Protein Deficits" (J. Brožek, ed.) pp. 255–269. DHEW Pub. No. (NIH) 79–1906.

30. Super, C., Clement, J., Vuori, L., Christiansen, N., Mora, J., and Herrera, M. G. (1981). Infant and caretaker behaviour as mediators of nutritional and social intervention in barriers of Bogota. *In* "Culture and Early Intervention" (T. Feild, A. Sostek, P. Vietze and P. Leidermann, eds) pp. 171–188, Lawrence Earlbaum, New Jersey.

31. Freeman, H. E., Klein, R. E., Townsend, J. W. and Leghtig, A. (1980). Nutrition and cognitive development among rural Guatemalan children. *Am. J. Publ. Hlth* **70**, 1277–1285.

32. Klein, R. (1979). Malnutrition and human behaviour: a backward glance at an ongoing longitudinal study. *In* "Malnutrition, Environment and Behaviour" (D. A. Levitsky, ed.) pp. 219–237. Cornell University Press, Ithaca and London.

33. Chavez, A. and Martinez, C. (1982). Neurological maturation and performance on mental tests. *In* "Growing Up in a Developing Community." Instituto Nacional de la Nutricion, San Fernando y Viaducto Ilalpan, Mexico.

34. Evans, D., Hansen, J. D. L., Moodie, A. D. and VanderSpuy, H. I. J. (1980). Intellectual development and nutrition. *J. Pediat.* **97**, 358–368.

35. Hicks, L. E., Longham, R. A. and Takenaka, J. (1982). Cognitive and health measures following early nutritional supplementation. A sibling study. *Am. J. Publ. Hlth* **72**, 1110–1118.

36. Mora, J. O., Amezquita, A., Castro, L., Christiansen, J., Clement-Murphy, J., Cobbs, L. F., Cremer, H. D., Dragastin, S., Elias, M. F., Franklin, D., Herrera, M. G., Ortiz, N., Pardo, F., de Paraedes, B., Ramos, C., Riley, R., Rodriquez, H., Vuori-Christiansen, L., Wagner, M and Stare, F. J. (1974). Nutrition, health and social factors related to intellectual performance. *In* "World Review of Nutrition Dietetics," Vol. 19, pp. 205–236. S. Karger, Basel.

37. McKay, H. E., McKay, A. and Sinisterra, L. (1973). Behavioural intervention studies with malnourished children: a review of experiences. *In* "Nutrition Development and Social Behaviour" (D. J. Kallen, ed.) pp. 121–146. DHEW Pub. No. (NIH) 73–242.

38. Sinisterra, L., McKay, H., McKay, A., Gomez, H. and Korgi, J. (1979). Response of malnourished preschool children to multidisciplinary intervention. *In* "Behavioural Effects of Energy and Protein Deficits" (J. Brožek, ed.) pp. 229–238. DHEW Pub. No. (NIH) 79–1906.

39. Kielmann, A. A., DeSweemer, C., Blot, W., Vberoi, I. S., Robertson, A. D. and Taylor, C. E. (1983). Impact on child growth, nutrition and psychomotor development. *In* "Child and Maternal Health Services in Rural India: The

Narangwal Experiment" (C. E. Taylor and R. Faruquee, eds) Vol. 1, Integrated Nutrition and Health Care, pp. 95–125. A. A. Kielmann and Associates: A World Bank Research Publication.
40. Monckeberg, F. (1968). Effect of early marasmic malnutrition on subsequent physical and psychological development. *In* "Malnutrition, Learning, and Behaviour" (N. S. Scrimshaw and J. E. Gordon, eds) pp. 267–269. MIT Press, Cambridge, Massachusetts.
41. Grantham-McGregor, S. M. (1984). Rehabilitation after clinical malnutrition. *In* "Malnutrition and Behaviour: A Critical Assessment of Key Issues" (J. Brožek and B. Schürch, eds) p. 531–554. Nestlé Foundation, Lausanne, Switzerland.
42. Yatkin, U. S. and McLaren, D. S. (1970). The behavioural development of infants recovering from severe malnutrition. *J. Ment. Def. Res.* **14**, 25–32.
43. Cravioto, J. (1977). Not by bread alone: effect of early malnutrition and stimuli deprivation on mental development. *In* "Perspectives in Pediatrics" (O.P. Ghai, ed.) pp. 87–104. Interprint, New Delhi.
44. Monckeberg, F. (1979). Recovery of severely malnourished infants: Effects of early sensory-affective stimulation: *In* "Behavioural Effects of Energy and Protein Deficits" (J. Brodzek, ed.) pp. 121–130. DHEW (NIH) Publ. No. 79–1906.
45. Celedon, J. M. and De Andraca, (1979). Psychomotor development during treatment of severely marasmic infants. *Early Human Dev.* **3**, 267–275.
46. Celedon, J. M., Csaszar, D., Middleton, J. and De Andraca, I. (1980). The effect of treatment on mental and psychomotor development of marasmic infants according to age of admission. *J. Ment. Def. Res.* **24**, 27–35.
47. McLaren, D. S., Yatkin, Y. S., Kannawati, A. A., Sabbagh, S. and Kadi, Z. (1973). The subsequent mental and physical development of rehabilitated marasmic infants. *J. Ment. Def. Res.* **17**, 173–181.
48. Cravioto, J. and Arrieta, R. (1979). Stimulation and mental development of malnourished infants. *Lancet* **ii**, 899.
49. Grantham-McGregor, S., Stewart, M. and Schofield, W. (1980). Effect of long term psychosocial stimulation on mental development of severely malnourished children. *Lancet* **ii**, 785–789.
50. Grantham-McGregor, S. M., Schofield, W. and Harris, L. (1983). Stimulation on mental development of severely malnourished children: an interim report. *Pediat.* **72**, 239–243.
51. Grantham-McGregor, S. M., Schofield, W. and Powell, C. (1987). The development of severely malnourished children who received psychosocial stimulation: Six year follow-up. *Pediat.* **79**, 247–254.
52. Rao, D. H. and Naidu, A. N. (1977). Nutritional supplementation—whom does it benefit most? *Am. J. Clin. Nutr.* **30**, 1612–1616.
53. Martorell, R., Lechtig, A., Yarbrough, C., Delgado, H. and Klein. R. E. (1976). Protein–calorie supplementation and postnatal physical growth: a review of findings from developing countries. *Arch. Lat. Nutr.* **XXVI**, (2), 115–128.
54. Martorell, R. and Klein, R. (1980). Food supplementation and growth rates in preschool children. *Nutr. Rep. Int.* **21**, 447–454.
55. Gopalan, C., Swaminathan, M. C., Kuman, V. K. K., Rao, D. H. and Vijayaraghavan, K. (1973). Effect of calorie supplementation on growth of undernourished children. *Am. J. Clin. Nutr.* **26**, 563–566.
56. Mora, J. O., Sellers, S. G., Guescun, J. and Herrera, M. G. (1981). The impact of supplementary feeding and home education on physical growth of disadvantaged children. *Nutr. Res.* **1**, 213–225.

57. Pollitt, E. (1980). Poverty and malnutrition in Latin America. *In* "Early Childhood Intervention Programs: A Report to the Ford Foundation," Praeger Special Studies. Praeger Scientific, New York.

58. Grantham-McGregor, S. M. and Desai, P. (1975). A home-visiting intervention programme with Jamaican mothers and children. *Dev. Med. Child Neurol.* **17**, 605–613.

59. Darlington, R. B., Royce, J. M., Snipper, A. S., Murray, H. W. and Lazar, I. (1980). Preschool programs and later school competence of children from low-income families. *Science* **208**, 202–205.

60. Beaton, G. H. and Hossein, G. (1982). Supplementary feeding programs for young children in developing countries. *Am. J. Clin. Nutr.* **35** (Suppl).

61. Sellers, S. G., Mora, J. O., Super, C. M. and Herrera, M. G. (1982). The effects of nutritional supplementation and home education on children's diets. *Nutr. Rep. Int.* **26**, 727–741.

62. Martorell, R., Klein, R. and Delgado, H. (1980). Improved nutrition and its effects on anthropometric indicators of nutritional status. *Nutr. Rep. Int.* **21**, 219–230.

63. Herrera, M. and Super, C. (1983). School performance and physical growth of underprivileged children: results of the Bogota project at seven years. Report to World Bank. Harvard School of Public Health, Cambridge, MA. As cited by Halpern, R. (in press). Effects of early childhood intervention on primary school progress and performance in Latin America. *Comp. Educ. Rev.*

64. McKay, A. and McKay, H. (1983). Primary school progress after preschool experience: troublesome issues in the conduct of follow-up research and findings from Cali, Columbia Study. Meyers, R. (eds.) *In* "Preventing School Failure: The Relationship Between Preschool and Primary Education" (K. King and R. Meyers, eds). International Developmen Research Center, Ottawa.

65. Chavez, A. and Martinez, C. (1981). School performance of supplemented and unsupplemented children from a poor rural area. *In* "Nutrition in Health and Disease and International Development," pp. 393–402. Alan, Liss, New York.

66. Berrueta-Clement, J. R., Schweinhart, L. J., Barnett, W. S., Epstein, A. S. and Weikart, D. (1984). "Changed Lives. The Effects of the Perry Preschool Program on Youths Through Age 19. The High/Scope Press, Michigan.

Acknowledgements

The Jamaican studies referred to in this paper were funded by the Ford Foundation, Overseas Development Administration and the Wellcome Trust, UK. I thank M. H. N. Golden for reading the manuscript.

Commentary

Linda S. Crnic: Before commenting on specific points, I shall make some more general comments. These were the first of the contributions to the

Workshop which I read. They provoked in me a feeling of impatience with
the lack of progress in this field and a sadness and sense of frustration. I
would agree with Grantham-McGregor that the uncontrolled research
described in her paper should stop, and I would go a step farther and suggest
that we may have reached the point of diminishing returns even in carefully
controlled studies in this area of research. This type of research is a
tremendous effort, and those who do it well are to be commended for their
heroic efforts. Grantham-McGregor reviews methodological issues in this
research, and her review serves to emphasize the great difficulty in achieving
adequate experimental design to permit clear conclusions from being drawn
from the data. The research on this topic, as good as some of it is, has served
mostly to define the parameters of the problem, and has achieved few
solutions and answered few questions. Let me be clear that defining the
parameters of the problem has been an exceedingly useful enterprise. As a
result of this research, we have a very clear picture of the complexity of the
problem and the complexity of solutions to the problem. This has had and
will continue to have important effects upon intervention strategies, even
if we cannot answer academic questions about causality. What we must
consider is that some of the questions about causality may never be answerable
in human, and perhaps not even in animal studies. This is due, in part, to
the fact that in both cases, the effects of nutrition and environment are
inextricably entwined.

I bring up the issue of diminishing returns in human field studies in order
to be constructive; that is, I hope to provoke a reconsideration of the goals
and design of such studies. One issue which arose, but went unanswered in
our discussion, is whether it would be profitable to design studies to compare
interventions. There are those who would argue that this is dangerous when
we have not solved the question of the true relationship between nutrition
and environment in causing the adverse outcomes. An additional suggestion
for the design of human field studies is to make use of the latest techniques
devised by developmental psychologists to assess performance. The
profitability of such a strategy is well illustrated in Barrett's work. This is
not a particularly easy undertaking because it is necessary to obtain the
cooperation of a developmental psychologist who is willing and able to adapt
his or her measures to the culture of interest. However, I believe that this
is an extremely efficient strategy which will improve the validity of the
measures used.

At least a part of my sadness engendered by reading this paper relates to
a more general issue. Much of medical research is aimed at determining the
causes of disorders and at devising cures for those disorders. In the case of
the effects of malnutrition, both the cause and cure is known. It is thus
distressing that such tremendous effort is expended to study the problem.

The sadness comes from the fact that we live in a world where the elimination of suffering and poverty in children is not enough to motivate governments to take action. It seems we must prove that this suffering warps their brains in order to justify intervention. Thus, while the cause and prevention of malnutrition is known, we do not know how to alter the political structure to bring about prevention.

One of the most important advances in this field has been the realization that malnutrition does not operate in a vacuum, but is accompanied by other physical ills (e.g. infection) and usually an environment which is suboptimal for development. A further realization which seems to be slow in coming is that of the interactive nature of the relationship between a child and her environment. As Grantham-McGregor has emphasized in her research [1], the child must not be viewed as an independent actor, rather than as part of a mother–infant unit. She makes the interesting point that feeding an entire family may lead family members to treat the index child differently. The nutritional status of either member of a dyad will influence the behaviour of both members, because one's behaviour is in part a response to the behaviour of the other member of the dyad. In this way, as has been shown in animals (reviewed in 2), the malnourished child has a different environment than normal by virtue of his or her own behaviour [3].

Grantham-McGregor cites some animal research on the effects of environmental stimulation in remediating the effects of malnutrition. This is an area in which better use could be made of the animal data. This data can be used to ask how environmental stimulation has its effect, namely, does it reverse the effects of malnutrition or does it provide the organism with experiences which enable it to find alternative ways of solving problems? The answer, at this time, from animal research is that both mechanisms must be used: some neurochemical [4–6], neuroanatomical and brain weight [7–15] parameters can be ameliorated by environmental stimulation, some cannot [4–14]. When behaviour is normalized while gross measures of biochemical composition of the brain remain abnormal [16], it is likely that environmental stimulation provides the organism with the flexibility to use alternative strategies for solving behavioural problems in the face of brain deficits.

1. Grantham-McGregor, S. M. (1984). Social background of childhood malnutrition. *In* "Malnutrition Behavior: A Critical Assessment of Key Issues" (J. Brožek and B. Schürch, eds) pp. 358–372. Nestlé Foundation, Lausanne, Switzerland.
2. Crnic, L. S. (1984). Nutrition and mental development. *Am. J. Ment. Def.* **88**, 526–533.
3. Chavez, A. and Martinez, C. (1975). Nutrition and development of children from poor rural areas. *Nutr. Rep. Int.* **11**, 477.
4. Cines, B. M. and Winick, M. (1979). Behavioural and psysiological effects of early handling and early malnutrition in rats. *Devl. Psychobiol.* **12**, 381–389.

5. Eckert, C. D., Levitsky, D. A. and Barnes, R. H. (1975). Postnatal stimulation: The effects on cholinergic enzyme activity in undernourished rats. *Proc. Soc. Exp. Biol. Med.* **149**, 860–863.
6. Morgan, B. L. G. and Winick, M. (1980). Effects of environmental stimulation on brain N-acetylneuraminic acid content and behavior. *J. Nutr.* **110**, 425–432.
7. Bhide, P. G. and Bedi, K. S. (1982). The effects of environmental diversity on well-fed and previously undernourished rats: I. Body and brain measurements. *J. Comp. Neurol.* **207**, 403–409.
8. Bhide, P. G. and Bedi, K. S. (1984). The effects of a lengthy period of environmental diversity on well-fed and previously undernourished rats. I. Neurons and glial cells. *J. Comp. Neurol.* **227**, 296–304.
9. Bhide, P. G. and Bedi, K. S. (1984). The effects of environmental diversity on well fed and previously undernourished rats: neuronal and glial cell measurements in the visual cortex (area 17). *J. Anat.* **138**, 447–461.
10. Davies, C. A. and Katz, H. B. (1983). The comparative effects of early-life undernutrition and subsequent differential environmental on the dendritic branching of pyramidal cells in rat visual cortex. *J. Comp. Neurol.* **218**, 345–350.
11. Katz, H. B. and Davies, C. A. (1982). The effects of early-life undernutrition and subsequent environmental on morphological parameters of the rat brain. *Behav. Brain Res.* **5**, 53–64.
12. Katz, H. B. and Davies, C. A. (1983). The separate and combined effects of early undernutrition and environmental complexity at different ages on cerebral measures in rats. *Devl. Psychobiol.* **16**, 47–58.
13. Katz, H. B., Davies, C. A. and Dobbing, J. (1980). The effect of environmental stimulation on brain weight in previously undernourished rats. *Behav. Brain Res.* **1**, 445–449.
14. Katz, H. B., Davies, C. A. and Dobbing, J. (1982). Effects of undernutrition at different ages early in life and later environmental complexity on parameters of cerebrum and hippocampus in rats. *J. Nutr.* **112**, 1362–1368.
15. Sara, V. R., King, T. L. and Lazarus, L. (1976). The influence of early nutrition and environmental rearing on brain growth and behavior. *Experientia* **32**, 1538–1540.
16. Crnic, L. S. (1983). Effects of nutrition and environment on brain biochemistry and behavior. *Devl. Psychobiol.* **16**, 129–145.

J. Dobbing: I would like to agree with Crnic that "we may have reached the point of diminishing returns even in carefully controlled (field) studies in this area of research". I do not believe that analytical techniques, or experimental or survey designs exist, nor are likely to be devised, which will add much to what we already know about the extraordinary complexity of factors in the environment, perhaps including nutrition, which help to shape an individual's future achievement (1). I believe that to continue to indulge in variants of the field-study methods merely to re-iterate what we have already learned from them, that we should feed children, is a mis-use of research funding. Experimental studies can still be justified, since they could still help us understand the advisability of humanitarian aid at certain vulnerable periods in a child's development; and for some they are justified purely for their scientific value. The same cannot, in my view, any longer be pretended for the field studies on humans.

1. Dobbing, J. (1985). Infant nutrition and later achievement. *Am. J. Clin. Nutr.* **41**, 477–484.

S. A. Richardson: I believe that we need to ask why the topic of the long-term consequences of undernutrition in infancy has instigated so many studies and so many reviews of studies. The reasons why the topic has aroused sustained international interest may provide a perspective and focus for evaluating the research in malnutrition. As a starting point, I would like to ask why all this research in malnutrition has been carried out and to what extent have the questions that were originally posed been answered.

One major factor that led to interest in the long-term effects of undernutrition was advances in medical treatment around the mid-twentieth century which made it possible to keep alive children who would earlier have died as the result of severe malnutrition. Physicians responsible for the care of severely malnourished children then became concerned that they might be saving children who, as the result of malnutrition, had permanent damage to the central nervous system, which would cause severe life-long impairment of intellectual functioning. If this proved to be the case, this would have profound implications for national policies and priorities in many parts of the world.

During the same period of time international relief agencies were publicizing the plight of starving people, and it was generally believed that severe malnutrition was widespread in developing countries. The high proportion of beds in hospitals in developing countries occupied by children with severe malnutrition was seen as evidence that malnutrition existed in similar proportions among children living in areas surrounding the hospitals. What may be called the famine model of malnutrition dominated most people's thinking, and it is unfortunate that the epidemiological question was not addressed of how prevalent was malnutrition in different countries? It was only recognized later that in many countries the famine model did not apply. Rather, in countries where there was no overall shortage of food, there was a low prevalence of malnutrition, but sufficient for them to be seen frequently in pediatric wards of hospitals. Had this been more widely recognized, it might have led to research into the causes of malnutrition in order to find methods of prevention. Instead, this question has been ignored, and the focus of research has been on the consequences of malnutrition.

The early research findings that infants who had suffered severe malnutrition functioned less well on intellectual tests than children who had not been malnourished appeared to confirm fears about the long-term damaging effects of malnutrition on intellectual development. These findings were widely promulgated and were used to give added urgency to international efforts to ship food to areas where there was evidence of malnutrition. The rationale of using the research findings was to use food to prevent malnutrition because; once malnourished, a child would suffer irreversible CNS damage with life-time intellectual impairment or mental retardation.

The need to prevent hunger and prevent malnutrition should be judged on humanitarian grounds. This seems self-evident, but given the opportunity to use the interpretation given to early research findings on the effects of malnutrition, the spectre of high rates of mental retardation was used as a reason for promoting food shipments to developing countries. By the late 1960s, the conventional wisdom at the international level was that malnutrition caused mental retardation, and this view was expressed by the news media, professionals, governmental and non-governmental organizations. This in turn stimulated expanded funding for studies of the consequences of malnutrition. The topic of malnutrition and its effects was added to research meetings dealing with mental retardation and still is a topic at such meetings.

The chapters in this volume by Smart, Barrett, Grantham-McGregor, Galler and Sinisterra make it clear that the original research conclusions were based on grossly inadequate designs and methods, and the conclusions drawn by the authors were unjustified. The follow-up studies of malnourished children largely ignored the wide array of factors which influence intellectual development, both social and biological. To expect to control all factors other than malnutrition that may influence the cognitive and social development of children by selecting controls matched on two or three variables, such as sibship or social class, seems ludicrous. There has been a shift in studies from simple, so-called "experimental" studies toward more complex conceptual models and designs which are more ecological and longitudinal. Some of these studies are reviewed by Grantham-McGregor. The studies which use an ecological model show that social experiences account for most of the differences found between children who were and were not malnourished and that the malnutrition, depending on the general context in which it occurs, has little or no direct influence. The study in Barbados (see chapter by Galler, this volume) is one of the most recent, and the author's conclusion is discrepant with previous studies. The results are interpreted as showing that early childhood malnutrition has a dominant effect on intellectual development and that the social environment and circumstances of upbringing have little effect. I believe these results should be subjected to critical evaluation to see whether the author's conclusions are justified.

The early interpretation of malnutrition studies separately carried out in follow-up studies of malnourished children, animal studies, and investigations of the brain had a joint impact in the development of the conventional wisdom that malnutrition in infancy causes mental retardation.

The present reviewers show that these conclusions were unjustified on scientific grounds and concur with a number of previous reviewers that there is still no clear evidence that malnutrition has any demonstrated long-term irreversible effects on intellectual and social development (1). If malnutrition has any effects, they are slight. There is still considerable opposition to this position, and this is not surprising, given how widespread and strong was the conventional wisdom about the effects of malnutrition.

If we return to the question originally posed by physicians, "Does severe malnutrition in infancy result in permanent and severe mental impairment for the individual?", the evidence from the present and reviews suggests a negative answer to the question. This conclusion in no way should detract from the goal of trying to eliminate hunger and famine in all countries in the world. Such a goal does not need the support of scientific findings on the long-term consequences of undernutrition.

We may ask, "What has been learned other than that the original fears and claims about the long-term effects of severe malnutrition were unwarranted?" I believe we have learned:

(1) Severe malnutrition in infancy does not condemn a child to severe irreversible intellectual impairment.

(2) Severe malnutrition in infancy, except in times of warfare, natural catastrophes, and general starvation, is usually found in the context of a general set of social and biological conditions that together place the child at severe disadvantage for intellectual and social development. The provision of better feeding alone, without attending to the wide range of other conditions that place the child at intellectual and social disadvantage, will be of little use. The conditions of disadvantage include those with which the child directly interacts, such as the family, but also include conditions which only affect the child indirectly and are mediated through the family, such as the general, physical, social, and economic conditions of the community, and the more general environments in which the child lives.

(3) A number of studies reviewed by Grantham-McGregor have contributed to our understanding of various forms of social intervention with families for the purpose of assisting the social and intellectual development of children. They have been shown to have some short-term effects, but there is as yet scant evidence of long-term beneficial effects for the child. These studies began in part to attempt

to overcome the lack of experiences provided for the social and emotional needs of the child in the hospital. Other studies appeared to be based on the premise that malnutrition had caused some intellectual impairment, and the intervention to provide intellectual stimulation was intended to counter the assumed damaging effects of the malnutrition. The benefits obtained for the children may well be unrelated to malnutrition, and the evidence of the studies needs to be considered in the broad context of the intellectual stimulation literature. Because experimental designs have been used, the investigators have neglected to examine whether differential effectiveness of the intervention within the experimental group was related to differences in the home and more general environmental conditions in which the experimental children lived. Social stimulation studies have some rationale in being focussed on malnourished children, because malnutrition is often an indicator of general disadvantage for the child. However, there are many children living in equally disadvantaged conditions who are not malnourished, but who would benefit as much from social stimulation and should be considered for inclusion.

(4) As long as malnutrition was thought to exist as the result of famine, warfare, or natural catastrophes, the focus of research attention was on the consequences of the malnutrition. In our own work in Jamaica and from other studies, it appears that malnutrition occurs under conditions where there is no widespread food shortage, and most children do not experience malnutrition. Under these conditions, the study of the circumstances, conditions, and mechanisms under which malnutrition occurs in infancy may provide valuable clues that may lead to some prevention.

(5) The research in malnutrition began because of concern about the intellectual and social development of children. This should be a primary concern of every society. It is this broad concern that demands research attention in the future, rather than the single possible etiological factor of malnutrition for later intellectual and social development.

(6) From an historical perspective, there are many examples of single factors that were claimed to be largely responsible for various impairments in children. In mental retardation, genetic factors were claimed to be the cause, and this position was widely supported internationally in the social movement of eugenics. Thirty years ago it was widely claimed by obstetricians that difficulties during the birth process were largely responsible for cerebral palsy and other congenital neurological defects. Perhaps the etiological role of malnutrition in impaired intellectual and social development of children will in the future be seen as another such example.

Grantham-McGregor points out the lack of care of investigators in defining the severity and duration of undernutrition of the children studied. I would add that there is rarely a rationale given for the kind of undernutrition that has been selected. In general, it seems reasonable when studying the effects of an entity, to study the entity first in its most severe form, in order to give the best chance of finding effects. If the extreme case shows clear effects, then it becomes worth studying the entity in more moderate forms. The same reasoning applies to duration of the entity, when it is postulated that duration may influence the effects.

Often reports of research do not specify what conceptual model was used in the study, and it has to be inferred. I believe it would be useful to review the various conceptual models that have been proposed. Perhaps the two that are most comprehensive are those of Cravioto *et al.* (2) and Chavez and Martinez (3). Both these models include the sequence of undernutrition, leading to infection, leading to reduced activity and stimulation, leading to impoverishing early experience, in turn leading to impairment of social and intellectual development. Within this sequence the relationship between undernutrition, immunization, and infection seem important. This topic has recently been reviewed by Chandra (4). Grantham-McGregor discusses some of the methodological problems of studies in which food supplements are given to the experimental group. I would add to these problems as follows:

(1) Food is intimately tied to customs, practices, habits, and beliefs. A change in food is likely to lead to chains of reaction that affect other aspects of living, making it difficult to use a food supplement without introducing other unintended consequences.

(2) There is an ethical problem of food supplements over time changing the ecology of food in the study community. The community may become dependent on the supplement and experience difficulties at the end of the study when food supplementation is terminated.

In the social stimulation studies reviewed by Grantham-McGregor, the forms of intervention are based on methods developed outside of the country where the intervention takes place. An alternative strategy would be to carry out careful field studies comparing the socialization practices, parental characteristics, and general conditions and history of the households in which children (a) do well in social and intellectual development, and (b) do poorly in social and intellectual development. From such studies, valuable information may be gained about practices which produce effective socialization within the local communities. Such practices may then provide valuable clues to forms of intervention which work locally and which are likely to be acceptable.

1. Richardson, S. A. (1984). The consequences of malnutrition for intellectual development. *In* "Scientific Studies in Mental Retardation" (J. Dobbing *et al.*, eds). Macmillan Press, London.
2. Cravioto, J., Birch, H. G., DeLicardie, E. R. and Rosales, L. (1967). The ecology of infant weight gain in a pre-industrial society. *Acta Paed. Scand.* **56**, 71–84.
3. Chavez, A. and Martinez, C. (1982). "Growing Up in a Developing Community". Instituto Nacional de la Nutricion, San Fernando y Viaducto Ilalpan, Mexico.
4. Chandra (1983). Nutrition, immunity and infection: present knowledge and future direction. *Lancet* 688.

J. Dobbing: I agree with the general sense of Richardson's remarks and have already set them out elsewhere (1). However, I cannot yet jump, as he does, from there being "still no clear evidence that malnutrition has any demonstrated long-term irreversible effects on intellectual development", to there being a "negative answer to the question". The possibility still exists, for me, that nutrition may play a part, amongst a host of other environmental influences, even though it probably cannot be conclusively demonstrated because of the complexity of the necessary measurements and analysis. Richardson correctly points out, as I have on many occasions, the fallacy of discussing the subject in terms of "brain damage" and "mental retardation" (1).

1. Dobbing, J. (1985). Infant nutrition and later achievement. *Am. J. Clin. Nutr.* **41**, 477–484.

I. Hurwitz: This survey report again catalogues the variety of methodological and design deficits which appear to be rampant in a whole host of studies which have attempted to document the relationship between early nutritional states and later "achievement", the latter term referring to a wide array of outcome performance including measures of intelligence and social and affective behaviours. I say "again" with respect to the shortcomings reported in these investigations, because these criticisms appear repeatedly in this paper and in papers recently published elsewhere (1) which deal with this same research question.

The specific problems centre on inadequate matching of control and experimental populations, the comparisons of projects carried out in different geographical settings whose populations have vastly different cultural and social mores despite their sharing membership in the "Third World" or as "developing nations", inadequate knowledge of the non-nutritional effects of supplementation, and the lack of measurement instruments genuinely appropriate to the populations and samples being studied.

Despite the somewhat less than encouraging overall picture which emerges, Grantham-McGregor's paper reports findings which, when taken in conjunction with the results of other studies, begin to show that whatever else may happen in the face of a variety of programmes of nutritional supplementation, improved environmental stimulation, and enhanced parent–child interaction for the very young child, produce effects which appear to emerge in an increase in motor competence, motor activity and fine and gross motor coordination. Summarizing the findings from studies in Colombia, Guatemala and Mexico, Grantham-McGregor finds that, "supplement was reported to favour the more motoric and manipulative skills, rather than linguistic and cognitive ones up 3 years of age," and further in the report, "the supplemented group showed a remarkable increase in activity levels and exploration. The mothers in turn showed more responsiveness to their supplemented children; this was interpreted to indicate that the more active exploring child invoked more stimulating behaviour in the mother". Similar findings are derived from pilot studies in Colombia ("reported to have increased activity levels"), India, ("higher scores on psychomotor testing in gross and fine motor development"), and so on.

It may be interesting to speculate on what the significance of increased or improved psychomotor progress in development may mean to different cultural groups. This is to say that it is conceivable that not every society regards increased physical activity as a positive characteristic in the young child. It may even be interpreted as a less than desirable characteristic. Such increased activity may affect the parent–child interaction adversely, and the subsequent effect may be to reduce the child's eagerness and enthusiasm for activity and exploration. In Western society it appears that a positive value is placed upon independence, separation, and individuation (2), albeit after an essential initial period of attachment or "bonding". However, the thrust of *positive* development appears to be in the direction of self-definition and autonomy, and this is achieved, ostensibly, at the earliest levels through motor activity, its development and refinement. Tied to this aspect of motor development is its perceived benefits in cognitive development, particularly in the earliest period defined by Piaget as the sensorimotor stage and even beyond, in the pre-operational and concrete operational phases (3). Thus, in those societies where motor competence is seen as a valued instrumentality of both social and emotional development, its enhancement through early nutritional supplementation with or without other forms of intervention will likely produce longer range beneficial effects as determined eventually by measures of psychological performance.

On the other hand, it has been observed that certain cultural groups in other than Western societies place a greater emphasis on prolonged periods of intimacy, closeness and/or attachment between mother and child, and that motor activity is seen as a centrifugal force which accelerates a process of separation which is in fact considered to be undesirable (4). One can speculate that in these circumstances the impact of nutritional supplementation on motor activity may have an adverse influence on the mother–child interaction, and that, while the observable effect may indeed be to increase "responsiveness", the nature, quality and above all the meaning of this increased responsiveness to both mother and child would have to be ascertained. In other words, observed outcomes need to be understood, not only in terms of values imposed from the researcher's own frame of reference, but it is essential that the culture or society be understood in its own socioecological terms. This may be a ponderously obvious comment, but one which I think has been underemphasized in the research literature on malnutrition and undernutrition.

Grantham-McGregor's own study of long-term psychosocial intervention in Jamaican children, which included play, home visits, introduction of toys, and *parent education and encouragement* (italics mine), demonstrated a clear improvement in language development, occurring earliest and maintaining its advantage over "locomotor" development throughout the study. As I understand this report, there was no component of nutritional supplementation, so that that factor, which has been reported elsewhere to have its effect on motor development, was absent, and the major, indeed exclusive rehabilitative report, was psychosocial stimulation which carried with it a heavy emphasis on "talking to and with the child", thus yielding the not surprising finding with respect to the differential outcomes between language and non-language areas. Furthermore, and here again I venture onto speculative terrain, I note that as an essentially Western society, Jamaica might very well follow the expected emphasis on language development and language usage as a positive cultural value, fostering distancing and individuation between parent and child. In the original article in fact, Grantham-McGregor does point out that the intervention programme did emphasize verbal communication in the type of stimulation provided to children and mothers.

The latter part of this paper carefully documents many of the specific methodological difficulties which intervention studies have demonstrated. These touched on such problems as randomization of assignment of cases, age at which supplementation is initiated, the timing of introduction of "psychosocial stimulation" as well as its duration, etc. In addressing the question of supplementation treatment and the enormous variability in the circumstances in which this type of programme is implemented, Grantham-McGregor concludes that "in those studies where neither growth nor dietary intake is reported, and there is no response in development, it is impossible to interpret the results of supplementation with any degree of certainty". Perhaps the most telling aspect of Grantham-McGregor's comments in the area of the effects of psychosocial stimulation is captured in her conjecture that the decline in gains over time in the Jamaica and Bogota studies, where home visits and parent instruction were involved, was related to the "impression that both mothers and visitors *wearied* (italics mine) of the performance towards the end". This is more, in my estimation, than a casual observation. Rather it emphasizes the need for programmes which, in addition to the educational, stimulation, and even nutritional elements they contain, must emphasize the enthusiasm, optimism, and energy which will maintain a high level of cooperativeness, interest, and sustained application. Nothing, it would seem, can be as corrosive to the long-term success of such stimulation programmes as the tendency for them to become boring, routinized and monotonous.

It is somewhat discouraging perhaps, despite the scattered patterns of reported improvements in IQ, motor activity, academic achievement and social behaviour, that information on mediating biological mechanisms and the persistence of inadequate research design make definitive conclusions on the roles and importance of various factors insufficient to generate genuinely effective programmes. It is a sobering fact to consider that in a review of studies as comprehensive as exists in this paper, only one, the Bogota research, can be identified as one which examined the effects of improving *both* nutritional and psychosocial conditions. The consequences of this is simply to drive home the fact that more sophisticated and meaningfully formulated studies have yet to be done to meet the world need for effective rehabilitative programmes.

1. Brožek J, and Schürch, B. (eds) (1984). "Malnutrition and Behavior: A Critical Assessment of Key Issues." Nestlé Foundation, Lausanne, Switzerland.
2. Mahler, M. (1975). "The Psychological Birth of the Human Infant." Basic Books, New York.
3. Piaget, J. and Inhelder, B. (1954). "The Construction of Reality in the Child." Basic Books, New York.
4. Spence, J. (1981). Presidential Address, American Psychological Association. Toronto.

J. L. Smart: One of the advantages of a workshop like this and the publication arising from it, is that it affords participants the opportunity to escape from the strait-jacket of routine scientific writing; the sort of writing we all do for journals, which is necessarily stereotyped, often conveys a mistaken impression of how the research was planned and organized, and is shorn of much that might be of interest. Happily, Grantham-McGregor has seized the chance to say something rather different. Her insights into the methodological problems of intervention studies in particular are perceptive and refreshingly frank. I cannot imagine anyone stating in a paper for a journal that (p. 146), "In Jamaica, we had the impression that both mothers and visitors wearied of the programme towards the end". This is not just interesting, it is important information with respect to the planning of future intervention programmes.

I should like to consider intervention, be it nutritional or otherwise, in relation to the characteristic, "learned helplessness". I suggested in my paper that some malnourished or formerly malnourished children may exhibit learned helplessness; that is, they may feel helpless to improve their lot and effectively give up. Of course, the parents of such children are quite likely to exhibit the same characteristic. It is possible that one of the indirect benefits of intervention may be to jolt the family out of the torpor of learned helplessness. By the very nature of the phenomenon, it is probably best overcome by therapy that rewards self-help or demonstrates the benefits of personal effort. Hence, enlisting the active participation of the parents in the rehabilitation of the child is likely to be more effective than hand-outs of food, health-care or even stimulation. The community health aides in Grantham-McGregor's study encouraged the mothers to become involved in stimulating their children and it may have been partly for this reason that the DQ/IQ levels of the stimulated group remained appreciably higher than those of non-stimulated index children for years after the cessation of the intervention programme (Fig. 1).

K. S. Bedi: The chapter by Grantham-McGregor reviews the now not inconsiderable literature related to the effects of undernutrition during early life on behavioural functioning in later life in humans. The point which stands out most clearly from the literature is that it is almost impossible to be sure that any deficits observed in behavioural performance are not due to the unavoidable presence of other environmental factors such as disease and social and physical deprivation, rather than due to the undernutrition. In other words, the people who suffer from a period of undernutrition are also those who have to endure poor education, housing and other adverse environmental conditions. This, and the fact that suitable controls are often not available, make it very difficult to separate from other complicating factors the effects in man of the level of nutrition.

Given these unavoidable complications, is it really any surprise that it has been impossible to obtain unequivocal answers to the important question of whether undernutrition during early life inhibits subsequent intellectual development? Even with improved methodological advances, surely it is *always* going to be impossible to control all the various environmental factors to which human populations are subject during their development. Humans simply do not make good "experimental" material for such studies. Unfortunately, animal studies can only ever provide evidence which is of indirect relevance to humans. We are therefore left with an insoluble dilemma.

An important question raised by the papers reviewed by Grantham-McGregor (and also considered by Sinisterra in his chapter) is whether or not a stimulating environment in later life can remove some of the behavioural deficits produced as a result of malnutrition during early life. This question is sufficiently distinct to be worthy of some comment. Grantham-McGregor reviews several papers which have purported to study this question in humans. None of them have been particularly satisfactory. For instance Winick and his colleagues (1) analysed the IQ scores of a sample of 6–12-year-old Korean girls, adopted before the age of three into middle class American homes. Records of height and weight were used to classify some of these girls as having been previously malnourished. Although such girls had persisting deficits in IQ when compared with the well-nourished group, they nevertheless had IQs not significantly different from the "mean of the US schoolchildren of the same age". The authors use this last fact to suggest that the "enriched" American environment has caused the "catch-up" in mental performance. Unfortunately the study lacked an important control: there were no previously malnourished girls placed in a poor environment to compare with those in the "enriched" environment. In addition, cultural factors which are capable of influencing IQ tests were not controlled in this study. Grantham-McGregor's chapter does not point out these shortcomings clearly.

The idea that the later environment may be able to modulate the effects of early life undernutrition has perhaps come from a series of studies on animals. There have been claims that environmental "enrichment" or "impoverishment" can cause alterations in brain growth, morphology, biochemical nature as well as in the behaviour of animals. The vast majority of these studies have been published by Rosenzweig and his associates (1) in America. There have also been some animal studies which have seemed to indicate that environmental stimulation can "normalise" the behaviour of nutritionally deprived rats (2,3).

Recent research conducted in this laboratory (4–8) has brought into question some of the previous claims, concerned with the possible morphological changes in the brains of environmentally enriched or impoverished animals. In addition in experiments (4–13) where both well fed and previously undernourished rats have been raised in either enriched or impoverished conditions, it has been found that there were no statistically significant interactions between nutrition and environment, even for those few features which appeared to show a main effect of environment. This indicates that undernutrition during early life does not preclude animals from interacting with their environment in a manner which can produce similar changes in brain morphology to those observed in normally nourished animals.

The implications of these observations for the management and treatment of malnourished children are speculative, but nevertheless of some importance. For instance, it may be heartening to predict from these results that children malnourished during early life should still be capable of responding to their environment in a manner which should produce similar changes in brain structure to those likely to be observed in well nourished children. However, the additional observation that the environment cannot completely, or even largely, restore many of the morphological deficits in the brain which result from undernutrition during early life must remain a matter of some considerable concern. One final caveat mentioned in my own chapter but re-emphasized now, is that with our present state of knowledge it is not possible to ascribe any particular morphological alteration to a given change in behaviour, even if this can be detected.

1. Winick, M., Meyer, K. K., and Harris, R. C. (1975). Malnutrition and environmental enrichment by early adoption. *Science* **109**, 1173–1175.
2. Rosenzweig, M. R. and Bennett, E. L. (1978). Experiential influences on brain anatomy and chemistry in rodents. *In* "Studies on the Development of Behaviour and the Nervous System: Early Influences" (G. Gottlieb, ed.) pp. 289–327. Academic Press, New York.
3. Franková, S. (1968). Nutritional and psychological factors in the development of spontaneous behaviour in the rat. *In* "Malnutrition, Learning and Behaviour" (N. S. Scrimshaw and J. E. Gordon, eds) pp. 312–322. MIT Press, Cambridge, MA.
4. Levitsky, D. A. and Barnes, R. H. (1972). Nutritional and environmental interactions in the behavioural development of the rat: long term effects. *Science* **176**, 68–71.
5. Bhide, P. G. and Bedi, K. S. (1982). The effects of environmental diversity on well fed and previously undernourished rats: Body and brain measurements. *J. Comp. Neurol.* **207**, 403–409.
6. Bhide, P. G. and Bedi, K. S. (1984). The effects of environmental diversity on well fed and previously undernourished rats: neuronal and glial cell measurements in the visual cortex (area 17). *J. Anat.* **138**, 447–462.
7. Bhide, P. G. and Bedi, K. S. (1984). The effects of a lengthy period of environmental diversity on well fed and previously undernourished rats. I. Neurons and glial cells. *J. Comp. Neurol.* **227**, 296–304.
8. Bhide, P. G. and Bedi, K. S. (1984). The effects of a lengthy period of environmental diversity on well fed and previously undernourished rats. II. Synapse-to-neuron ratios. *J. Comp. Neurol.* **227**, 305–310.
9. Katz, H. B., Davies, C. A. and Dobbing, J. (1980). The effects of environmental stimulation on brain weights in previously undernourished rats. *Behav. Brain Res.* **1**, 445–449.
10. Katz, H. B. and Davies, C. A. (1982). The effects of early life undernutrition and subsequent environment on morphological parameters of the rat brain. *Behav. Brain Res.* **5**, 53–64.

11. Katz, H. B., Davies, C. A. and Dobbing, J. (1982). Effects of undernutrition at different ages early in life and later environmental complexity on parameters of the cerebrum and hippocampus in rats. *J. Nutr.* **112**, 1362–1368.
12. Katz, H. B. and Davies, C. A. (1983). The separate and combined effects of undernutrition and environmental complexity at different ages on cerebral measures in rats. *Devl. Psychobiol.* **16**, 47–58.
13. Davies, C. A. and Katz, H. B. (1983). The comparative effects of early life undernutrition and subsequent differential environments on the dendritic branching of pyramidal cells in rat visual cortex. *J. Comp. Neurol.* **218**, 345–350.

D. E. Barrett: There are several aspects of Grantham-McGregor's presentation which concern me. These involve (a) insufficient attention to the question of whether or not the studies reported were based on a clear theoretical rationale, (b) dismissal of retrospective studies as not contributing to our understanding of the effects of undernutrition, and (c) failure to recognize that "inconsistencies" in results of supplementation studies may be due, in large part, to the fact that the studies have often addressed different questions.

(a) Grantham-McGregor reports results of studies on the effects of malnutrition with a critical eye to methodology, but not to theoretical rationale. Thus, when "negative" results are reported, there is no questioning of whether results may have failed to be identified because the researchers were not measuring the most relevant outcome variables. For example, Grantham-McGregor writes "The striking finding of *absolutely no effect of supplementation on mental development* (my italics) of undernourished 3-year-old children, in two studies in Cali, Colombia . . . may be associated with their somewhat older age". Is it possible that supplementation did affect the behaviour and "mental development" of the children but that sensitive indicators were not used to measure behavioural outcomes? (See my commentary on Sinisterra's chapter this volume.)

I have argued, both here in this Workshop and elsewhere (1), that we should be careful about concluding, after reviewing malnutrition studies showing "no effects on intellectual development", that malnutrition had no adverse effect on the child's behavioural development. In many studies, the researchers select outcome variables not on theoretical grounds but out of convenience, habit, or desire to make a social point (e.g., malnutrition does (or does not) permanently retard intellectual development). We should pay closest attention to studies in which the authors test a specific, theoretically justified hypothesis about the behavioural effects of malnutrition. The studies of Richardson and colleagues (2) and Galler and colleagues (3) illustrate appropriate theoretical derivation of outcome variables.

I would like to refer to our findings (4,5) in Guatemala on the effects of nutritional supplementation on children's social and emotional characteristics at school age. Across villages, there were effects of supplementation on attention, persistence, affect, play with peers, and interest in the physical environment. Except in one village, IQ effects were negligible. However, IQ effects were not strongly predicted by our theoretical position. I would argue that the development and even the "mental development" of the subjects was influenced by their nutritional history, even in the absence of IQ effects.

(b) Grantham-McGregor says "that retrospective studies are, due to their methodological limitations, unlikely to clarify the nature of the relationship between severe malnutrition and mental development and should be discouraged." I believe that what Grantham-McGregor calls retrospective designs (and these are, specifically, designs in which data are collected retrospectively and the analysis is prospective, with group membership based on differences on the presumed antecedent variable (1,6)) address fundamentally different questions than do experimental designs, and may be very important to our understanding of malnutrition and behaviour.

I would like to quote from a recent chapter (7) in which I addressed this question:

When the central purpose of a study is an unequivocal identification of cause-effect relationships between malnutrition and behavior, an experimental design is necessary (p. 587). . . . But we should not assume that one type of design is best for all purposes.

A non-experimental design is appropriate when the purpose of the study is to examine and compare the contributions of several potential independent variables to variation in an outcome variable of interest *under the conditions in which these variables normally operate; i.e., allowing for the covariations between the independent variables present under natural circumstances.* Experimental designs negate natural dependencies between independent variables. This is, of course, the intent: by ensuring that individual differences in potentially confounding variables are randomized across treatments, they make it possible to infer that between-group differences result from the independent variable of interest (i.e., malnutrition or nutritional supplementation). However, in so doing, they are in effect asking the question "If the groups were comparable with respect to certain variables which we know to be or believe to be related to our outcome variable, then — under *these* conditions — what would be the effect of our treatment (i.e., improved nutrition) on the criterion variable?" However, it may be *precisely* the case that under natural conditions malnutrition exerts influence on a particular behavioral outcome only when it occurs in conjunction with other non-nutritional factors, and that, under other (e.g., the experimental) conditions, its potential contribution to behavior is moderated or offset. In such instances, the experimental manipulation may lead us to an inappropriate conclusion about the relationship between nutrition and behaviour in the population of interest. (p.588)

I believe that retrospective comparison studies are often the proper first step in the development of an experimental, nutritional intervention design.

(c) Grantham-McGregor reviews results of supplementation studies. She notes, correctly, that subjects may respond differently to treatment, depending on initial nutritional status and dietary intake. She suggests that such differences may explain some of the inconsistencies.

Her summary statement on intervention studies is "It is apparent that both nutritional supplementation and stimulation affects development in some children in some circumstances. But in which subjects, with which types of treatment and to what extent, and whether there is an interaction between treatments remains uncertain".

I do not question the conclusion that the results of nutritional supplementation will depend on the above factors. But I think it is wrong to consider the differences in findings as "inconsistencies" and to imply, therefore, that the whole question of the effect of supplementation on behaviour is problematic.

I view the "inconsistencies" (what I would call apparent differences in findings) as due primarily to the fact that the studies are often addressing different research questions. The theoretical question of the effects of intervention X on a certain class of behaviour outcomes Y in an extremely malnourished population is a different one from the question of the effect of the same type of intervention on the same class of behaviour outcomes for a better-nourished population. The effects of a particular supplement in dose A for a duration of J years is a different question from the effects of the supplement in dose B for J years, or the effects of the supplement in dose A for K years.

It is a problem common in nutritional intervention research that the researcher fails to indicate, both in conceptualizing and reporting his research, what the target population was (i.e. to whom results may be generalized); to what "levels" of the construct the independent variable may be generalized (e.g. for all amounts of daily energy supplement or only for the range of 100–200 additional kcal per day); and what the precise nature of the independent variable is (i.e. nutritional supplementation alone or nutritional supplementation and a certain degree of social involvement with subjects). I have referred to these problems (1) as problems in the "construct validity of putative causes and effects". (The term is from Cook and Campbell (8).) The first problem is inadequate specification of the target population; the second is "confounding of the construct with level of the construct" (8); and the third is inadequate conceptualization of the independent (treatment) variable.

In reviewing the research studies, we should first ask what the specific research issue (in terms of type of supplement, amount of supplement, type of population, and criterion variables) was. We should expect differences in findings in studies which differ on these factors, and try to interpret the differences in terms of the specific theoretical questions which the different studies addressed. If we do this, we will find that the different findings are interpretable and not simply a mass of "inconsistent", problematic results.

1. Barrett, D. E. (1984). Methodological requirements for conceptually valid research studies on the behavioural effects of malnutrition. *In* "Nutrition and Behavior" (J. R. Galler, ed.) pp. 9–36. Plenum Press, New York.
2. Richardson, S. A., Birch, H. G., Brabie, E. and Yoder, K. (1972). The behavior of children who were severely malnourished in the first two years of life. *J. Biosoc. Sci.* **7**, 255–267.
3. Galler, J. R., Ramsey, F., Solimano, G., Lowell, W. E. and Mason, E. (1983). The influence of early malnutrition on subsequent behavioral development. II. Classroom behavior. *J. Am. Acad. Child Psych.* **22**, 16–22.
4. Barrett, D. E., Radke-Yarrow, M. and Klein R. E. (1982). Chronic malnutrition and child behavior: Effects of early caloric supplementation on social and emotional functioning at school age. *Devl. Psychol.* **18**, 541–556.
5. Barrett, D. E. and Radke-Yarrow, M. (1985). Effects of nutritional supplementation on children's responses to novel, frustrating and competitive situations. *Am. J. Clin. Nutr.* **42**, 102–120.
6. Fleiss, J. L. (1982). "Statistical Methods for Rates and Proportions", 2nd edn. John Wiley, New York.
7. Barrett, D. E. (1984). Methodological issues in nutritional intervention research. *In* "Malnutrition and Behavior: A Critical Assessment of Key Issues" (J. Brožek and B. Schürch, eds) pp. 585–596. Nestlé Foundation, Lausanne, Switzerland.
8. Cook, T. D. and Campbell, D. T. (1979). "Quasi-experimentation: Design and Analysis for Field Settings." Rand-McNally, New York.

D. A. Levitsky and Barbara J. Strupp: The review of field studies on the effects of early nutrition and stimulation provides a fairly broad outline of most of the major research in this area. Of particular importance is the author's good criticism of many of these studies on the basis of (a) study design, (b) the problem of taking psychological measurements in large field studies, (c) the selection of subjects, (d) small effects of nutritional supplementation, and (e) failure to provide a "mechanism" (theoretical framework) to explain the effects (or lack of effects) of environmental stimulation or nutritional supplementation.

However, this neglect of interest in theoretical mechanisms also applies to the author, as well as to the research she critisizes. For example, the author states: "Most studies which have failed to find associations between poor mental development and severe malnutrition have involved cases of kwashiorkor." This is an extremely interesting conclusion that is of considerable theoretical importance, but one which received no comment by the author. Its theoretical significance lies in the fact that many researchers (including the writers of this commentary) have been arguing for a long time that one of the mechanisms through which malnutrition affects human development is by producing behavioural and psychological responses that are incompatible with the normal acquisition of environmental information. Since it is commonly observed that children suffering from kwashiorkor appear to be more behaviourally disturbed than marasmic children, we would expect that children experiencing kwashiorkor would be *more* cognitively affected than marasmic children, not less affected. Clearly this problem deserves more attention.

In another vein, it is interesting to note that the title of the chapter, "Field Studies in Early Nutrition and Later Achievement", refers only to nutrition as the independent variable. Yet, the author devotes much of her chapter to the discussion of the use of environmental stimulation as an adjunct to nutritional rehabilitation. In fact, the author's general conclusion is that "both nutritional supplementation and stimulation affect development in children" demonstrates the major importance that Grantham-McGregor applies to the interaction between the two variables and suggests that each alone is not sufficient to produce long-term gains in achievement.

But what are the mechanisms? And why are the long-term effects so poor? Perhaps if we had a better theoretical understanding of what is being affected by malnutrition and of the role played by early environment in cognitive development, we might be better able to answer some of these questions than we are at present.

J. Dobbing: One thing that strikes me about the chapters written for this Workshop on "field studies" is that none of them make very much (or indeed any) appeal or reference to the biology of the matter. Does this mean that they do not see the relevance of it? Are their interests solely in observational studies, and do they not see any of their conclusions having a biological basis? Or are their interests in behavioural outcome conditioned by a conscious belief that the brain has nothing to do with them? If so they could, of course, be right, in the same sense that my criticism of much of what I see as deficient in a television programme can have nothing to do with the television receiver.

That being said, I think that all three "field studies" chapters (those by Grantham-McGregor, Galler and Sinisterra, this volume) are weakest where they approach biology, for example in talking about the science of nutrition, with which I am bound to say they seem to have little acquaintance! All three are clear that nutrition is only one of a host of other environmental variables, but none of them ask very clearly whether it is a relevant variable at all; still less do they give any place to the important trilogy of developmental nutrition: its timing in relation to age, its severity, or its duration. So perhaps it is even further from our subject, in their view, to ask them to consider the brain as part of the organ of thought?

The Interaction of Nutrition and Environment in Behavioural Development

JANINA R. GALLER

*Center for Behavioural Development
and Mental Retardation, Boston University School of Medicine,
Boston, MA, USA*

Introduction

In the modern era of more effective promotion of health for the prevention and treatment of diseases in developing regions of the world, an increasing population of survivors of early malnutrition has emerged. Because of this, the focus during the past twenty years has shifted from efforts to reduce the high infant morbidity and mortality rates in these parts of the world to a increasing concern with the later effects of malnutrition. The majority of studies has evaluated physical growth and development following malnutrition. However, the importance of intellectual and behavioural functions has also been recognized.

This chapter will first review available studies on the long-term consequences of early malnutrition. This will be followed by a section identifying the variety of environmental factors which play a part in generating the state of malnutrition and in determining its sequelae. Finally, a discussion of the principles of analysis applied to this problem will complete the chapter.

Early Nutrition and Later Achievement
ISBN: 0-12-218855-1

Long-term Consequences of Malnutrition

The available studies of the long-term effects of malnutrition on behaviour can be broadly categorized into those that are *retrospective (cross-sectional)* and *longitudinal* in design. Each of these types of study has advantages and limitations, which are discussed briefly below. *Retrospective studies* have been performed at one point in time and data from earlier points in time were inferred, or gathered by questioning or review of records. Examples of such studies include those by Cravioto and his colleagues in Guatemala in 1966 (12) testing intersensory integration or the ability to transfer from one sensory modality to another among 143 short and tall rural and 120 short and tall urban children aged 6–11 years. The highest number of errors on the test battery was recorded for the short rural children presumed to have been chronically malnourished from early childhood on the basis of growth failure. Clearly, a major disadvantage of this type of research is the imprecision associated with identifying earlier events which contributed to the current state of function. However, in many circumstances, retrospective studies provide information which could not be easily obtained otherwise. In the Guatemalan study, a much larger population of children would have been required at birth to obtain a sample of 243 children with different degrees of undernutrition due to high infant mortality rates and migration in these communities.

In another more recent retrospective study, Winick and his colleagues (41,57) studied IQ and school achievement in 240 Korean schoolgirls who had been adopted by American families at five years of age or below. Retrospective diagnosis of severe and moderate malnutrition and adequate nutrition by review of height percentiles at the time of adoption allowed these authors to conclude that there were significant performance deficits among the children in the severely malnourished group, especially among those who were adopted at older ages and who had therefore presumably been exposed to longer periods of poor nutrition. In both the above studies, current height was used as a marker of preceding nutritional history without precise information about their early history. Nevertheless this approach has value because (a) it can be performed rapidly and inexpensively, and (b) it points to problem areas such as delayed verbal and intellectual skills which could be profitably studied in longer term investigations of recovery from malnutrition.

Longitudinal studies have examined subjects on more than one occasion, generally over an extended period of time. Such studies have advantages over retrospective studies in that they allow the evaluation of causal relationships between an earlier event and later outcome, and allow the evaluation of the extent to which measurements early in life are predictive of later function.

However, they are also costly and subject to biases arising from changes over time in study conditions such as subject attrition, staff changes, environmental changes and conceptual changes in data collection and analysis (see 29 for a review of the application of longitudinal designs). Despite these limitations, longitudinal studies have provided the bulk of evidence for permanent behavioural deficits following an episode of malnutrition early in life. All of these studies have followed children *after* they were diagnosed with malnutrition.

Behavioural outcome after a history of infantile malnutrition has been studied through school age, and in some instances, through adolescence. Research on these long-term effects has focussed on various indices of intelligence and behaviour, including school performance (see 22 for an extensive review of this subject). Although the earliest studies compared children to local standards (for example, Cabak and Najdanvic (8) in Yugoslavia), this review will address only studies using control groups. These included ten studies, namely those by Liang *et al.* (40) in Indonesia, Evans *et al.* (19,20) in South Africa, Stoch and Smythe (52–54) and Stoch *et al.* (55) in South Africa, Champakam *et al.* (9) in India, Hertzig *et al.* (35) and Richardson *et al.* (48–50) in Jamaica, Birch *et al.* (5) and Cravioto and DeLicardie (14) in Mexico, Fisher *et al.* (21) in Zambia, Hoorweg and Stanfield (36,37) in Uganda, Pereira *et al.* (45) in India, and Galler *et al.* (23–27) in Barbados. There are also five longitudinal studies of children with early malnutritiion resulting from organic disease, namely cystic fibrosis or pyloric stenosis (Lloyd-Still *et al.* (42,43) and Beardslee *et al.* (1) in the United States, Klein *et al.* (39) in the United States, Berglund and Rabo (2) in Sweden, Valman (56) in England, and Ellis and Hill (18) in Canada).

In research on the long-term effects of infantile malnutrition on IQ and behavioural development, by far the most commonly studied indicator has been IQ. The usefulness of the IQ tests in such studies is limited. First, the tests may not be equally appropriate across different cultures and ethnic groups. Second, the clinical significance of an IQ deficit is not always clear in the absence of other information about a child's performance. Therefore, it is also necessary to examine other aspects of behavioural function that may also have bearing on the child's adaptive capabilities, such as school performance and behaviour in school.

Although conditions in each study vary widely, the results of longitudinal research on the sequelae of early malnutrition are generally consistent in demonstrating reduced IQ performance. Later IQ scores of children with a history of kwashiorkor were examined in five studies, four of which confirm deficits (Champakam *et al.* (9); Pereira *et al.* (45); Birch *et al.* (5); Galler *et al.* (27a)). In contrast, Evans *et al.* (19) and Hansen *et al.* (34) found no differences in IQ on the New South African Individual Intelligence scale (NSAIIS) between 40 South African children and their siblings, but they did find deficits in the malnourished group on the Harris–Goodenough reflecting emotional immaturity. In a recent intervention study by the same authors (20), dietary supplementation was provided to younger children of families having at least one older child diagnosed with kwashiorkor. These authors reported higher IQ scores in the supplemented children than in older siblings who either were or were not previously malnourished. This suggests that the older siblings who were used as a control group in the first set of studies were also undernourished and had IQ performance which was also reduced relative to South African standards.

The IQ of children with histories of marasmus was evaluated in two studies, both of which showed deficits. Stoch and Smythe (53,54) reported lower scores, especially in boys, on the NSAIIS in 20 South African children who were compared to controls matched for socioeconomic level. Galler *et al.* (23,27) found lower IQ scores in 129 Barbadian boys and girls with histories of marasmus who were compared at ages 5–11 and again four years later with 129 classmates and neighbourhood children who were well-nourished. In a more recent study, Galler and her colleagues (27a) directly compared intellectual performance in children up to 18 years of age with histories of kwashiorkor or marasmus during the first year of life. These authors found the same degree of impairment in the two previously malnourished groups on a variety of indices. The four remaining longitudinal studies include mixed cases of malnutrition, and these also confirm deficits in IQ among the previously malnourished children. Liang *et al.* (40), Hoorweg and Stanfield (36,37), and Fisher *et al.* (21) attribute these findings to the episode of severe malnutrition. However, Richardson *et al.* (50), in their study of 74 Jamaican schoolboys, their siblings, and well-nourished controls, concluded that deficits in IQ and other behavioural indices in their population resulted from the interaction of early malnutrition and a disadvantaged home environment.

In contrast to studies performed in developing regions of the world, studies of malnutrition secondary to medical illness which were undertaken in Western countries generally do not show IQ deficits. Thus, Ellis and Hill (18) studied "malnourished" and "well-nourished" children who had been diagnosed with cystic fibrosis, and Lloyd-Still *et al.* (42,43) and Beardslee *et al.* (1) studied children with cystic fibrosis up to 22 years of age using sibling controls. All reported no deficits in IQ in their small samples of previously malnourished children. In another study, Berglund and Rabo (2) found no association between IQ at the time of induction into the military and the severity of malnutrition in 180 Swedish men, all of whom had histories of pyloric stenosis. Unfortunately, there was no control group used in this latter study. Klein *et al.* (39), in the only study of this group with an adequate research design, compared 50 boys and girls, aged 5–14 years, having histories of pyloric stenosis, with 44 siblings and 50 adequately nourished controls. These authors found deficits suggesting impaired attention and short-term memory only in the malnourished group. Since they found no overall IQ deficits, they suggest that performance on specific IQ subscales should be evaluated. Although evidence from these studies has been used to demonstrate that early malnutrition *per se* has only a limited effect on IQ as distinct from disadvantaged environmental conditions, this conclusion is not justified. There are too few studies, based on small sample sizes, and for the most part there are major limitations in the selection of control groups. The most comprehensive study of this series, that of Klein *et al.* (39), does demonstrate persistent behavioural deficits, in conflict with the other studies.

In addition to IQ, *intersensory integration*, or the ability to transfer information from one sensory modality to another, has also been studied in previously malnourished children. Deficits in intersensory integration have been implicated in reading and writing disabilities (Birch and Lefford (4); Birch and Belmont (3)). Studies in India by Champakam *et al.* (9) and Pereira *et al.* (45), and in Mexico by Cravioto and DeLicardie (13,14) report deficits in intersensory integration among children with previous malnutrition.

A number of studies of the later effects of early malnutrition have directly examined *school performance*, including academic achievement and classroom behaviour. Five longitudinal studies by Evans *et al.* (19), Richardson *et al.* (48,49), Pereira *et al.* (45), Stoch *et al.* (55), and Galler *et al.* (24,25) report deficits in school performance in children with previous marasmus or kwashiorkor. As was the case with IQ, available evidence from studies of children with malnutrition resulting from organic illness fails to establish any consistent impairment in school achievement in these children (1,18,56).

Several studies have also evaluated behaviour in the classroom, which may be more closely related to school success or failure than IQ (25). Richardson *et al.* (48,49) reported reduced attention span, conduct problems, and limited social skills in previously malnourished Jamaican boys compared to both siblings and well-nourished classmates. Galler *et al.* (24) expanded these findings to girls and reported an increased incidence of attention-deficit disorder from 15% to 60% and deficits in social skills in both boys and girls with previous malnutrition. Klein *et al.* (39), in their study of children with histories of pyloric stenosis, report immaturity and hyperactivity in addition to reduced attention span and memory skills.

In summary, following an episode of early malnutrition, deficits in IQ and behaviour have been documented to be present at least as late as adolescence. The majority of longitudinal studies of children in developing countries report reduced IQ and school performance in previously malnourished groups.

Several studies also report aberrant classroom behaviour, specifically attention-deficit disorder, which may explain the greater incidence of school failure in these groups. These outcomes are fairly consistent regardless of the type of malnutrition: kwashiorkor, marasmus, or mixed types. The majority of studies of malnutrition secondary to organic illness do not show later deficits. However, these studies have serious limitations in research design, including small numbers of subjects and inadequate comparison groups, and therefore do not permit any conclusions to be drawn. The role of disadvantaged environmental conditions in these findings is discussed in the next section.

The Role of Environmental Factors

Most studies of the long-term effects of malnutrition have been performed in developing countries where this condition is severe and prevalent. Inquiry into the relationship between malnutrition and behaviour in these regions of the world has been complicated by the fact that malnourished children most often come from the lowest socioeconomic classes of the population. When impaired intellectual performance is documented in these children, there has been a tendency to oversimplify this relationship and to attribute behavioural deficits either primarily to nutritional factors without taking adequate account of environmental factors, or to environmental factors alone. These factors are not easily separated and may have contributed in several ways. First, disadvantaged circumstances such as poor sanitation and high rates of infection may lead to malnutrition (46). Second, once malnutrition has been established, environmental factors may exacerbate and prolong the episode. Finally, after the episode has subsided, the continuation of poor environmental conditions may contribute to impaired growth and intellectual development, both independently and interacting with poor nutrition.

In the human condition, the larger social matrix within which a child lives must be considered. Figure 1 shows the range of environmental conditions that, when seriously compromised, put a child at special risk for developing malnutrition and for a poor behavioural outcome. Each of the factors is affected by macroenvironmental features which characterize the socioeconomic class of the family, including income level, quality of housing, schooling, health care and other support services. Pavenstadt (44) and Bradley and Caldwell (7) have demonstrated that families within a given socioeconomic group differ widely in their home environment in terms of the kinds and amount of stimulation provided to children and the level of parental education. Thus, as shown in the figure, the specific family environment, including such factors as family size, composition and stability,

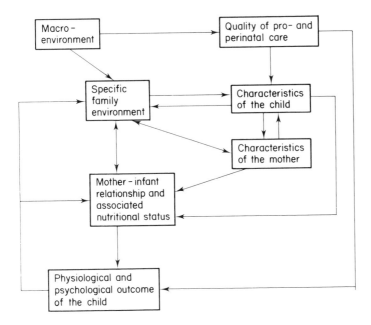

Fig. 1. Range of environmental conditions affecting the nutritional status and psychological outcome of the child. From (28).

may vary considerably within a specific socioeconomic group and predispose to and influence the outcome of malnutrition in the child. Characteristics of the child himself play a major role in this picture. Children who are of low birth weight, handicapped or sickly may be at greatest risk for developing malnutrition. Recently, temperament, or the child's innate character, has also been recognized to play a major role in modifying his response to adverse environmental conditions including malnutrition (17). Maternal characteristics, such as intelligence, social skills and psychological profile, may also serve to modify her response to her infant. Family, maternal and child characteristics determine or modify the synchrony of interaction between mother and child as measured by the pattern of mutual responsiveness of one to the subtle cues of the other over time. It should be noted that these factors are not specific to malnutrition, but have also been implicated in other childhood disorders stemming from a social origin. Furthermore, it is increasingly recognized that the relationship between disadvantaged environmental conditions and malnutrition is not a simple one. Rather, these are intricately intertwined throughout a child's development and influence his physiological and psychological outcome in concert.

This is illustrated in the following discussion of the available evidence concerning nutritional disorders and impairment of the mother–infant relationship.

The most persuasive evidence for differences among families that may lead to infantile malnutrition comes from the prospective study of Cravioto and DeLicardie (15,16) in Mexico. This study, which is the only prospective assessment of environmental conditions that predict malnutrition, concludes that deficits can be identified in the home that are antecedent to clinical malnutrition. These investigators followed 334 infants born in one year in a poor rural village; 22 of these children developed severe malnutrition (primarily kwashiorkor) some time in the first three years of life. These 22 children were then compared with 22 well-nourished children from the same cohort, who were matched according to birth weight and developmental quotient. The families of the two groups did not differ in terms of socio-economic features, including literacy, family size, parental age, or education, except that control families listened to radios more often.

The Caldwell Home Scale (Bradley and Caldwell, 7) was used to assess the home environments of the children *prior to* the episode of malnutrition; this technique relies on observation of the home and a structured interview with the mother or primary caregiver. Homes of children who would develop malnutrition were found to have lower scores in the quantity and quality of social, emotional, and cognitive stimulation available to the infant than did the homes of the control children. Additional observations of mother and infant during monthly developmental testing sessions in the first year of life indicated that mothers of the 22 malnourished children were less interested in their children's performance, less responsive, less sensitive to the children's needs, less verbally communicative, and less emotionally involved than control mothers.

Since the Mexican study by Cravioto and DeLicardie is the only systematic study of conditions in the home antecedent to the development of malnutrition, it is difficult to generalize without additional studies in other cultures. The other studies of mother–infant interaction are *concurrent with* or following an episode of malnutrition. As seen in other conditions of biological impairment (6), responses to the malnourished infant may be characterized by an *increased* amount of physical contact and suckling. In two well-designed and clearly presented studies, Graves evaluated patterns of mother–infant interaction in children with current undernutrition. Working in rural West Bengal, India (32) and in Katmandu, Nepal (33), Graves made 20-min observations of mothers and their infants of 7–8 months of age who had been identified in health clinics as being either moderately malnourished or well-nourished on the basis of anthropometric measures. In both studies, the malnourished infants showed low levels of play and spontaneous interaction with their mothers when they were in physical contact ("attachment behaviours"). However, malnourished infants spent significantly *more* time suckling at the breast and had more physical contact with their mothers than did comparison children.

These results also provided evidence for *cultural differences* in patterns of mother–infant interaction under conditions of malnutrition. Maternal behaviour differed in the two cultural settings. In India, mothers of malnourished infants initiated significantly less interaction with their infants as compared with mothers of the well-nourished children; in Nepal, there was no difference between the two groups.

Chavez and Martinez (11), working in a Mexican village, support these observations. These investigators provided nutritional supplementation to mothers and infants at risk for developing malnutrition. Not only did the supplemented infants and toddlers show improvement in physical growth and development, but also the mother–infant interaction was different from that in unsupplemented children (who were undernourished). Mothers of supplemented children were less overprotective and provided more opportunities for exploration and independence. For example, mothers of supplemented children spent 20% of the time in direct physical contact with their children as compared to 50% for mothers of non-supplemented children up to three years of age. Most of this time was spent in nursing. Such increased contact thus appears to be a common response to current malnutrition.

In a recent study in Jamaica, Grantham-McGregor and her colleagues (30,51) used the Caldwell Home Scale to assess home environment. Eighteen infants hospitalized for clinical malnutrition between the ages of 6 and 24 months of age were compared with a group of 21 adequately nourished children hospitalized for other reasons. Mothers of both groups of children were visited regularly at home beginning one month after the child's release from the hospital and up to 36 months later. The home environments of the two groups in this study were not found to be significantly different on the Home Scale. In contrast, Cravioto and DeLicardie found lower scores for homes of malnourished children up to 58 months of age in their study in Mexico. In addition, Grantham-McGregor and her co-workers also found that mothers of the malnourished children had lower verbal IQ scores than control mothers, whereas the Mexican study did not show this. Again, cultural differences in child-rearing patterns may have accounted for the diverging results. Two other studies have a bearing on the variable effects of malnutrition on the mother–infant interaction either at the time of the episode or later. One study in Jamaica, with very limited data, is that of Kerr *et al.* (38), who reported that severely malnourished children were more likely to come from unstable homes. In another study in the United States, Chase and Martin (10) compared with small groups of previously malnourished and well-nourished children who were matched in socioeconomic background, when they had attained 2–7 years of age. They found low scores on a home inventory scale, but no deficits in maternal IQ in the previously malnourished group.

Thus, the studies of concurrent responses to malnutrition do not present a unified picture. This is due in part to the use of different approaches to evaluating home environments. Three of the studies (11,32,33) made direct observations of the mother–infant relationship, and the others (10,15,16,30,38,51) used scales to score the quality of the home environment. In addition, within each group of studies there is evidence of culturally determined patterns of mother–infant interaction. Overall, these studies do not support the general assumption that malnutrition is associated with inadequate mothering. The one prospective study of Cravioto and DeLicardie does reflect this conclusion, but requires replication in other cultural settings. In two studies of children with malnutrition, there is evidence that suggests that changes in mother–infant interaction may actually compensate for the effects of the malnutrition. Thus, both Graves and Chavez reported increased physical contact with the mother and increased suckling in malnourished children. These responses may be a way to compensate for the child's malnutrition and the resultant biological impairment and may thus be protective of the malnourished child at the time of the malnutrition. It is possible that these concurrent responses to malnutrition are modified by inadequacies in the home environment, which were apparently present prior to the onset of malnutrition in at least two of the studies described.

In summary, many characteristics of the later home environment of a child with a history of early malnutrition may have been present earlier in life, contributing to the occurrence of the disorder and complicating the child's ability to recover from it. Nevertheless, only a limited number of studies of the long-term effects of early malnutrition have addressed this issue in detail.

Evaluating the Relative Contribution of Environment

The contribution of the variations in the home environment to the long-term consequences of infantile malnutrition remains an important but controversial issue. There are many methodological problems that face the wary investigator undertaking such longitudinal studies.

(1) What factors should be documented and how extensively?
(2) How should the extremely complex interactions between home environment and the early history of malnutrition be analysed as they affect the later behavioural outcome of the child?

(3) How can the life-long contribution of these factors be evaluated from early in the life of the child until maturity has been achieved?

We have addressed some of these matters in our studies of the long-term effects of early protein–energy malnutrition on the growth and mental development of Barbadian schoolchildren, and these are discussed in the following section.

Briefly, at the time of our studies, Barbados had a National Nutrition Centre, which identified all cases of infantile and childhood malnutrition and provided a service of health visitors and nutrition counsellors to correct the subsequent nutritional and health status of the child up to 11 years of age. Consequently, this provided an ideal setting for studying the long-term effects of early malnutrition uncomplicated by continuing inadequacies in the diet.

From this population, we have followed nearly all the children born between 1967 and 1972 who developed moderate to severe malnutrition in the first year of life. From the excellent hospital obstetric records, it was possible to standardize this group by including only those children with normal birth weights, uneventful perinatal periods, and no encephalopathic events during childhood, thus excluding other factors with potential negative effects on later development. This population yielded 129 children with histories of protein–energy malnutrition characterized by weight loss to a level below 75% of expected weight for age, muscle wasting and loss of subcutaneous fat. To these children, we matched 129 classmates without any history of malnutrition who were of similar age and sex and from the same socioeconomic group. All children were surveyed extensively at three points during their school years from 5 to 18 years of age at which time 85% of the original population was still available for study. To these two groups of children were applied a battery of tests of growth and development, cognitive function, cognitive performance (IQ, soft neurological signs, Piaget's tests of conservation) and behaviour, and an evaluation of environmental conditions early in life and at later ages.

Range of Environmental Factors

No study can include all possible environmental factors which affect childhood development. Therefore, a selective appraisal of the literature dealing with disadvantaged children and their mental function during childhood provides the basis for the identification of a range of environmental variables which have been implicated as contributory to aberrant outcomes of these children. This approach was applied by Richardson (47) in his study of 74 Jamaican schoolchildren with histories of infantile malnutrition, and was adopted by us in our study of the long-term effects of malnutrition in Barbados. Factors which emerged in both studies were as follows: (a) *biological characteristics* of the mother, including reproductive, health and nutritional history; (b) *maternal characteristics*, including her social interactions, verbal abilities, and educational achievement; (c) *father's characteristics*, including his presence in the home, educational level, and degree of agreement with his wife regarding childrearing; (d) *family size and composition*; (e) *child's experience* in the family, including the number of caretakers, amount of stimulation available such as story telling, books and games in the home, and the child's relationship with adults and other children; (f) *physical and economic resources*, including number and type of home conveniences, income and food expenditure, type of household, employment and means of transportation. The range of environmental factors used in different studies and the need for developing uniform and reliable measures of social background in studies of malnutrition has recently been emphasized in a review by Grantham-McGregor (31).

Testing the Interaction Between Nutrition and Environment

The first step of any analysis is to produce, from a given data set, a limited number of variables which can comprehensively describe the social environment of a given child. There are many acceptable techniques of data reduction which can be applied, including *a priori* grouping of items into a set number of categories, or more sophisticated analytical techniques. In our study of Barbadian schoolchildren, we have elected to apply factor analysis to the data which statistically groups all related items into categories, known as factors. The relative contribution of each item to the overall schema is expressed as a *factor score*, which can be easily utilized in further statistical analysis of the data. An important advantage of data reduction in general is that it eliminates random findings which can result from the analysis of too many individual items.

Applying these techniques to the range of environmental conditions listed in the previous section, we identified seven factors describing the environmental conditions in families of children in our study. A comparison of factor scores between children with histories of protein–energy malnutrition and healthy comparison children from the neighbourhood who were classmates showed that, despite matching of the two groups, there were significant differences between them on five of the seven environmental factors, including home conveniences, family stability, type of transportation used, the child's experience in the home and mother's fund of knowledge. This at once raises the question, if the malnourished children were from a more disadvantaged background, was this the cause of their intellectual disabilities or was it malnutrition?

The next step was the measurement of the relative contributions of the environmental conditions and the history of malnutrition to later behavioural outcome. This statistical model took into account the possible interaction between malnutrition and environment, namely that certain environmental conditions may mitigate or augment the effects of malnutrition. In addition, the occurrence of malnutrition may be more frequent under certain disadvantaged environmental conditions and therefore environmental factors could be highly correlated with the history of malnutrition. To analyse the major factors influencing the IQ deficit observed in the Barbadian children with previous malnutrition, we created a 2×2 matrix in which the control group and malnourished group were each classified into those subjects with higher environmental scores and those with inferior environmental scores. This was done by creating an overall score for each group, based on the seven environmental factors tested, and then determining the median for *each* group. As shown in Table 1, the comparison children had significantly better mean IQ performance on the Full Scale test than children with previous malnutrition. However, neither category of child showed different IQs due to environmental classification. This was further examined by dividing IQ into verbal and performance tests. As Table 1 shows, there was a significant effect of environment restricted to the Performance IQ in both groups. This implies that Performance IQ was influenced by environmental factors irrespective of nutritional history.

Table 1. IQ scores of children with histories of malnutrition and comparisons classified by environmental scores falling above and below the median for each group.

	Index	Comparison	ANOVA[a]
Full Scale IQ:			
Above median	91	104	Nutrition: $F(1, 241) = 38 \cdot 9^b$
Below median	90	102	
Verbal IQ:			
Above median	99	112	Nutrition: $F(1, 241) = 45 \cdot 2^b$
Below median	98	110	
Performance IQ:			
Above median	84	97	Nutrition: $F(1, 241) = 29 \cdot 7^b$
Below median	81	92	Environment: $F(1, 241) = 4 \cdot 0^c$

[a] ANOVA: analysis of variance. [b] $p < 0 \cdot 001$. [c] $0 \cdot 05$.

These findings were further confirmed and amplified by multivariate analysis of this data (23,26). This procedure allows for testing the effect of one set of factors such as environment or nutritional history, while controlling for the other. From these analyses we conclude that nutrition and current environment can both influence the child's intellectual attainment. However, in our study each factor operated independently, the major contributor being the previous nutrition and associated conditions early in the life of the child (see below).

It is significant that in our analysis of attention deficit disorder in Barbadian children with previous malnutrition, environment was also shown to play a role. However, the previous malnutrition again dominated the incidence of the syndrome (24,26).

In other situations, a different relationship between current environment and malnutrition may emerge, as demonstrated by Richardson, Hertzig and Birch's earlier study in Jamaica (49,50). Two apparent reasons for the contrasting experiences emerge. First, the Barbadian cohort was enrolled in a follow-up intervention programme at the National Nutrition Centre extending up to 11 years of age, which may have prevented the full impact of the environment affecting outcome. Second, the socioeconomic status of the Barbadian population was much less variable and at a higher level than in Jamaica. This conclusion is that the role of environment in studies of malnutrition may vary, thus further emphasizing the need for comprehensive evaluation of this condition.

Retrospective Prediction of Environmental Status

A major unresolved problem in evaluating the role of the environment in longitudinal studies is that the assessment is restricted to a narrow window in the life of the individual. The use of this method assumes that families will remain in the same social status over extended periods, including early childhood.

In our study of Barbadian children, we have the unique advantage of continuous monitoring of the children from age 5 to age 18, and can therefore test the stability of the environmental factors. We find that the environmental factors were highly correlated over time (27), indicating that families of children in our study retain the same relative position. This implies that during the school years, the home learning environment was adequately described by the measurement we applied. This does not, however, imply a lack of change. In fact, all groups improved in socioeconomic status and the previously malnourished group more so than the others. This also implies that, early in childhood, the groups may have been even further apart. This includes deficiencies in mother–infant interaction and in other early environmental conditions.

The resolution of this problem eventually resides in a *total* longitudinal study from birth onwards prior to the onset of malnutrition. However, such a study clearly has ethical limitations. In our own study, these considerations lead us to conclude that the *early* histories of the children, including environmental factors leading to the episode of malnutrition, were the dominant contributors to later mental outcome. These are not readily separable in the early years.

Conclusion

The role of the environment has still to be finally assessed. It is unlikely that a single universal conclusion can be drawn which is applicable to all populations, since the relative severity of malnutrition and degree of environmental variation are not uniform in deprived populations. This emphasizes the importance of including environmental measures in future studies. Knowledge of environmental conditions accompanying malnutrition is also likely to facilitate appropriate interventions both at the time of illness and later.

References

1. Beardslee, W. R., Wolff, A. H., Hurwitz, I., Parikh, B and Shwachman, H. (1982). The effects of infantile malnutrition on behavioral development: A follow-up study. *Am. J. Clin. Nutr.* **35**, 1437–1441.
2. Berglund, G. and Rabo, E. (1973). A long-term follow-up investigation of patients with hypertrophic pyloric stenosis with special reference to the physical and mental development. *Acta Paediatr. Scand.* **62**, 125–129.
3. Birch, H. G. and Belmont, L. (1964). Auditory–visual integration in normal and retarded readers *Am. J. Orthopsychiatry* **34**, 852–861.
4. Birch, H. G. and Lefford A. (1964). Two strategies for studying perception in "brain damaged" children. *In* "Brain Damage in Children" (H. G. Birch, ed.) p. 46. Williams and Wilkins, Baltimore.
5. Birch, H. G., Pineiro, C., Alcalde, E., Toca, T. and Cravioto, J. (1971). Relation of kwashiorkor in early childhood and intelligence at school age. *Pediat. Res.* **5**, 579–585.
6. Boles, G. (1959). Personality factors in mothers of cerebral palsied children. *Genet. Psychol. Mongr.* **59**, 159–218.
7. Bradley, R. H. and Caldwell, B. M. (1977). Home observations for measurement of the environment: A validation study of screening efficiency. *Am. J. Ment. Def.* **81**, 416–420.
8. Cabak, V. and Najdanvic, R. (1965). Effect of undernutrition in early life on physical and mental development. *Arch. Dis. Child.* **40**, 432–534.
9. Champakam, S., Srikantia, S. and Gopalan, C. (1968). Kwashiorkor and mental development. *Am. J. Clin. Nutr.* **21**, 844–852.
10. Chase, H. P. and Martin, H. P. (1970). Undernutrition and child development. *New Engl. J. Med.* **282**, 933–939.
11. Chavez, A. and Martinez, C. (1975). Nutrition and development of children from poor rural areas. V. Nutrition and behavioural development. *Nutr. Rep. Int.* **11**(6), 477–489.

12. Cravioto, J., DeLicardie, E. R. and Birch, H. G. (1966). Nutrition, growth an neurointegrative development: an experimental and ecologic study. *Pediat.* **38**(2) (Pt.I), 319–372.
13. Cravioto, J. and DeLicardie, E. R. (1970). Mental performance in school age children. *Am. J. Dis. Child.* **120**, 404–416.
14. Cravioto, J. and DeLicardie, E. (1971). Infantile malnutrition and later learning. *In* "Progress in Human Nutrition" (S. Margan and N. Wilson, eds) pp. 80–96. AVI, Westport, CT.
15. Cravioto, J. and DeLicardie, E. (1972). Environmental correlates of severe clinical malnutrition and language development in survivors from kwashiorkor or marasmus. *In* "Nutrition, the Nervous System and Behavior", pp. 73–94. PAHO Publication No. 251.
16. Cravioto, J. and DeLicardie, E. R. (1976). Microenvironmental factors in severe protein–energy malnutrition. *In* "Nutrition and Agricultural Development: Significance and Potential for the Tropics" (N. S. Scrimshaw and M. Behar, eds) pp. 25–35. Plenum Press, New York.
17. deVries, M. W. (1984). Temperament and infant mortality among the Masai of East Africa. *Am. J. Psychiat.* **141**, 1189–1194.
18. Ellis, C. E. and Hill, D. E. (1975). Growth, intelligence and school performance in children with cystic fibrosis who have had an episode of malnutrition during infancy. *J. Pediatr.* **87**, 565–568.
19. Evans, D. E., Moodie, A. D. and Hansen, J. D. L. (1971). Kwashiorkor and intellectual development. *S. Afr. Med. J.* **45**, 1414–1426.
20. Evans, D., Bowie, M. D., Hansen, J. D. L., Moodie, A. D. and van der Spuy, H. I. J. (1980). Intellectual development and nutrition. *J. Pediatr.* **87**, 355–363.
21. Fisher, M. M., Killeross, M. C., Simonsson, M. and Elgie, K. A. (1972). Malnutrition and reasoning ability in Zambian school children. *Trans. R. Soc. Trop. Med. Hyg.* **66**, 471–478.
22. Galler, J. R. (1984). The behavioral consequences of malnutrition in early life. *In* "Human Nutrition: A Comprehensive Treatise" (J. Galler, ed.) Vol. V. Plenum Press, New York.
23. Galler, J. R., Ramsey, F., Solimano, G., Lowell, W. E. and Mason, E. (1983). The influence of early malnutrition on subsequent behavioral development. I. Degree of impairment in intellectual performance. *J. Am. Acad. Child Psychiatry* **22**, 8–15.
24. Galler, J. R., Ramsey, F., Solimano, G. and Lowell, W. E. (1983). The influence of early malnutrition on subsequent behavioral development. II. Classroom behavior. *J. Am. Acad. Child Psychiatry* **22**, 16–22.
25. Galler, J. R., Ramsey, F. and Solimano, G. (1984). The influence of early malnutrition on subsequent behavioral development. III. Learning disabilities as a sequel to malnutrition. *Pediat. Res.* **18**, 309–313.
26. Galler, J. R. and Ramsey, F. (1985). The influence of early malnutrition on subsequent behavioral development. VI. The role of the microenvironment of the household. *Nutr. Behav.* **2**, 161–173.
27. Galler, J. R., Ramsey, F. and Ford, V. (1986). A follow-up study of the influence of early malnutrition on development. IV. Intellectual performance in adolescence. *Nutr. Behav.* **3**, 211–222.
27a. Galler, J. R., Ramsey, F., Salt, P. and Archer, E. (1987). The long-term effects of early kwashiorkor compared with marasmus. II. Intellectual performance. *Ped. Gastro. Nutr.* (in press).

28. Galler, J. R., Ricciuti, H., Crawford, M. and Kucharski L. T. (1984). The role of mother–infant interaction in nutritional disorders. *In* "Human Nutrition: A Comprehensive Treatise" (J. Galler, ed.) Vol. V. Plenum Press, New York.
29. Goldstein, H. (1979). "The Design and Analysis of Longitudinal Studies". Academic Press, London.
30. Grantham-McGregor, S. M. and Stewart, M. E. (1980). The relationship between hospitalization, social background, severe protein–energy malnutrition and mental development in young Jamaican children. *Ecol. Food Nutr.* **9**, 151–156.
31. Grantham-McGregor, S. M. (1984). Social background of childhood malnutrition". *In* "Malnutrition and Behavior: Critical Assessment of Key Issues" (J. Brožek and B. Schürch, eds) pp. 358–372. Nestlé Foundation, Lausanne, Switzerland.
32. Graves, P. L. (1976). Nutrition, infant behavior and maternal characteristics, a pilot study in West Bengal, India. *Am. J. Clin. Nutr.* **29**, 305–319.
33. Graves, P. L. (1978). Nutritional and infant behavior: A replication study in Katmandu Valley, Nepal. *Am. J. Clin. Nutr.* **31**, 541–551.
34. Hansen, J. P. L., Freesman, C., Moodie, A. D. and Evans, D. E. (1971). What does nutritional growth retardation mean? *Pediat.* **47**, 299–313.
35. Hertzig, M. E., Birch, H. G., Richardson, S. A. and Tizard, J. (1972). Intellectual levels of schoolchildren severely malnourished during the first two years of life. *Pediat.* **49**, 814–824.
36. Hoorweg, J. and Stanfield, P. (1972). The influence of malnutrition on psychologic and neurologic development: Preliminary communication. *In* "Nutrition, the Nervous System and Behavior", pp. 55–63. PAHO Publication No. 251.
37. Hoorweg, J. and Stanfield, P. (1976). The effect of protein energy malnutrition in early childhood on intellectual and motor abilities in later childhood and adolescence. *Dev. Med. Child Neurol.* **18**, 330–350.
38. Kerr, M. A., Begues, J. L. and Kerr, D. S. (1978). Psychosocial functioning of mothers of malnourished children. *Pediat.* **62**, 778–784.
39. Klein, P. S., Forbes, G. B. and Nadar, P. R. (1975). Effects of starvation in infancy (pyloric stenosis) on subsequent learning abilities. *J. Pediat.* **87**, 8–15.
40. Liang, P. H., Hie, T. T., Jan, O. H. and Giok, L. T. (1967). Evaluation of mental development in relation to early malnutrition. *Am. J. Clin. Nutr.* **20**, 1290–1294.
41. Lien, N. M., Meyer, K. K. and Winick, M. (1977). Early malnutrition and "late" adoption: a study of their effects on the development of Korean orphans adopted into American families. *Am. J. Clin. Nutr.* **30**, 1734–1739.
42. Lloyd-Still, J. D., Wolff, P. H., Hurwitz, I. and Shwachman, H. (1974). Studies on intellectual development after severe malnutrition in infancy in cystic fibrosis and other intestinal lesions. *In* "Proceedings of the 9th International Congress on Nutrition" Mexico, 1972, Vol. 2, pp. 357–364. S. Karger, Basel.
43. Lloyd-Still, J. D., Hurwitz, I. and Shwachman, H. (1974). Intellectual development after severe malnutrition in infancy. *Pediat.* **43**, 306–311.
44. Pavenstadt, E. (1965). A comparison of child rearing environment of upper-lower and very low-lower class families. *Am. J. Orthopsychiatry* **35**, 89–98.
45. Pereira, S. M., Sundararaj, R. and Begum, A. (1979). Physical growth and neurointegrative performance of survivors of protein–energy malnutrition. *Brit. J. Nutr.* **42**, 165–171.
46. Ricciuti, H. N. (1981). Developmental consequences of malnutrition in early childhood. *In* "The Uncommon Child" (M. Lewis and L. A. Rosenblum, eds), pp. 151–172. Plenum Press, New York.

47. Richardson, S. A. (1974). The background histories of schoolchildren severely malnourished in infancy. *In* "Advances in Pediatrics 21" (I. Schulman, ed.), pp. 167–192. Medical Yearbook Publishers, Chicago.
48. Richardson, S. A. (1972). The behavior of children in school who were severely malnourished in the first two years of life. *J. Hlth Soc. Behav.* **13**, 276–284.
49. Richardson, S. A., Birch, H. G. and Hertwig, M. E. (1973). School performance of children who were severely malnourished in infancy. *Am. J. Ment. Def.* **77**, 623–637.
50. Richardson, S. A., Koller, H., Katz, M. and Albert, K. (1978). The contributions of differing degrees of acute and chronic malnutrition to the intellectual development of Jamaican boys. *Early Human Dev.* **2**, 163–170.
51. Sheffer, M. L., Grantham-McGregor, S. M. and Ismail, S. J. (1981). The social intervention of malnourished children compared with that of other children in Jamaica. *J. Biosoc. Sci.* **13**, 19–30.
52. Stoch, M. B. and Smythe, P. M. (1963). Does undernutrition during infancy inhibit brain growth and subsequent intellectual development? *Arch. Dis. Child.* **38**, 546–552.
53. Stoch, M. B. and Smythe, P. M. (1967). The effect of undernutrition during infancy on subsequent growth and intellectual development. *S. Afr. Med. J.* **41**, 1027.
54. Stoch, M. B. and Smythe, P. M. (1976). 15-Year developmental study on effects of severe undernutrition during infancy on subsequent physical growth and intellectual functioning. *Arch. Dis. Child.* **51**, 327–336.
55. Stoch, M. B., Smythe, T. M., Moodie, A. D. and Bradshaw, D. (1982). Psychosocial outcome and CT findings after growth undernourishment during infancy: a twenty-year developmental study. *Dev. Med. Child Neurol.* **24**, 419–436.
56. Valman, H. B. (1974). Intelligence after malnutrition caused by neonatal resection in ileum. *Lancet* **i**, 425–427.
57. Winick, M., Meger, K. K. and Harris, R. C. (1975). Malnutrition and environmental enrichment by early adoption. *Science* **190**, 1173–1175.

Commentary

J. L. Smart: It is a characteristic of retrospective studies such as Galler's that the information on the independent variables is collected at different times, usually years apart. Nutritional status is thus inferred from the fact of being hospitalized for malnutrition in infancy or not, whereas socioeconomic status is estimated years later at the stage at which behaviour is assessed. The assumption that socioeconomic status remains stable over long periods of time is certainly questionable. These two independent variables, labelled nutrition and socioeconomic status, differ in other characteristics also. The experience of malnutrition is acute (requiring hospitalization) and occurs at a known age (though there may be a chronic component too), whereas the experience of being reared under any constellation of socioeconomic conditions is continuous, probably changing (sometimes erratically), and poorly defined. It seems to me that these differences pose considerable problems for any statistical analysis which assumes that these variables are strictly comparable.

Galler addresses the question of the stability of socioeconomic status in her section on "Retrospective Prediction of Environmental Status" and reassures us that environmental factors were highly correlated over time in her study. Since this evidence is not yet published (1), I cannot comment in an informed way on it. All I would say at this stage is that, depending on what contributed to "environmental status", it might be hard for it not to correlate statistically over time, by virtue of certain core characteristics (e.g. maternal attributes) remaining the same.

I was gratified as an animal experimenter to note a striking correspondence between man, or rather woman, and rat. Galler's conclusion that *increased mother–child contact appears to be a common response to current malnutrition* exactly parallels my own conclusion for undernourished rats (2). An explanation has been put forward to account for this phenomenon in the rat, based on a thermoregulatory theory of mother–young contact which suggests that the mother leaves her young when her ventral surface temperature exceeds a threshold level. An undernourished litter, of smaller mass than a well-fed litter, will heat the mother's ventrum more slowly and hence she will remain longer in contact with it. I shall not pretend that I think that this parsimonious explanation applies to human mother–child contact, but I offer two other possible explanations for increased contact in malnourished dyads. The first, which might also apply to rats, is that a malnourished infant is likely to be less mature than a well-fed child, and longer contact may be characteristic of younger infants. The second explanation is teleological and suggests that increased suckling may have the desirable effect of stimulating maximum milk production from a sub-optimal source.

1. Galler, J. R., Ramsey, F. and Ford, V. (1987). A follow-up study of the influence of early malnutrition on development. IV. Intellectual performance in adolescence. *Nutr. Behav.* (in press).
2. Smart, J. L. (1980). Attempts at equivalent care for well-fed and underfed offspring: are the problems appreciated? *Devl. Psychobiol.* **13**, 431–433.

S. A. Richardson: Galler, along with other investigators of undernutrition, use the terms socioeconomic, socioeconomic class or social class in describing the social environment of children (hereafter referred to as SES). In several studies, in which the only environmental measure used is SES, the inference is made that malnutrition causes later functional impairment. SES has also been used to select "controls". Because SES has such prominence in malnutrition studies it deserves careful scrutiny.

SES has been widely used in epidemiological and sociological studies in the UK, USA and European countries. In the USA Warner and Hollingshead developed a measure of SES which used three indicators: (1) occupation of head of household; (2) income; (3) education of parents. From these indicators they made a 5-point scale along the general dimension of poverty–affluence. In 1951 the British Registrar General developed a classification of social class based on the occupation of the head of the household. A number of occupations roughly comparable in social and economic terms were grouped together and five categories were formed ranging from unskilled manual to professional. The USA and British classifications are highly correlated. The classifications are sometimes reduced in number. For example, in Britain the two categories of manual and non-manual are used. In the USA three categories of "blue collar", "white collar" and "professional" are used (the latter is used in the Barbados study for the occupation of the father).

When the SES is used to classify large populations, it provides at least a high level abstraction that roughly distinguishes the styles of life of families, and it is most useful when the population is well distributed across the range of the scale. It should be emphasized that SES is a high-level abstraction and does not directly cause malnutrition.

The use of SES has very limited value in studies of malnutrition for the following reasons:

(1) The families of malnourished children are heavily over-represented at the lower end of the SES scale, giving little or no spread on the measure.

(2) When comparisons are selected who are not malnourished from classmates in school these children will also be heavily over-represented at the lower end of the SES scale.

(3) Within each broad category of SES there will be wide variability in the experiences, environments, and histories of children in families of the same SES.

(4) The concept of SES comes from a number of premises that are not valid. The measure assumes (a) that the child is brought up in a stable primary family with the biological parents, and (b) that the head of the household is a male who has steady employment in the same kind of job. These assumptions ignore the realities of unstable families, children being raised by a succession of caretakers who may be unemployed, ill, disabled, or retired, and that patterns of child rearing and family structure vary across cultures. Family instability is likely to be particularly common in the families with malnourished children.

For these reasons SES is a poor measure for malnutrition studies, and the only justification for its use is in the selection of comparisons to avoid comparing families at opposite ends of the SES scale. After selecting comparisons within or around some rough SES measure, there remains wide variation in the social experiences and history of children with the same SES classification.

Several investigators have used classmates at school, age and sex as matching variables in selecting what are often then called "controls". This is done in the Jamaica and Barbados studies. In the Jamaican study it then became a study objective to examine in what ways the experience and life histories of the malnourished children were similar or different from comparisons. In the Barbados study the selection of comparisons was "To control for the adverse conditions in the child's environment that may have contributed to the long term behavioural outcome . . ." (1)

This difference in perspective in the two studies led to a major focus in the Jamaican study on the background histories of the malnourished and comparison children and their upbringing without the kinds of assumptions made in the SES concept. Rather the attempt was made to determine who were the significant mothers in the histories of upbringing of each child.

The study in Barbados did not begin with field work to learn about the kinds of lives and histories of their study population and then develop measures appropriate to their particular population. Instead, they used an abbreviated and simplified set of the variables used in Jamaica and only obtained cross-sectional data on the current circumstances and conditions of the children at ages ranging from 5–11.

In the early reports of the Barbados study dealing with the influence of early malnutrition on subsequent behavioural development they found that current SES made little or no contribution to IQ, classroom behaviour, and learning disabilities. For the reasons that I have given this finding does not warrant the conclusion that the early history of malnutrition and its accompanying conditions are leading contributors to the later impairment.

In a later paper (Galler's reference 26) they use a stepwise multiple regression analyis (Table 5) to examine the correlation of classroom behaviour and IQ with nutritional history and a measure of the microenvironment of the family. "The result was . . . the nutritional history was still significantly correlated with the same four classroom behaviours and with IQ even when the environmental factors were controlled" (p. 168).

From these results they conclude:

> . . . that a poor microenvironment contributes to the precipitation of exacerbation of an episode of malnutrition, which in turn results in functional brain changes which express themselves as an attention deficit disorder and reduced IQ.

There are some reasons why this conclusion is not justified by the data and analysis used. First, they assume that the environmental measure obtained when the children's ages were 5–11 are the same environments that obtained around the time of malnutrition in infancy: "that many of the environmental factors observed by us at the time have persisted from early childhood and were instrumental in causing the episode of malnutrition" (p. 172).

Second, that the results were "significant" is based on their being significantly different from 0. In the table the highest R^2 values account for only 19% of the variance for full scale IQ and 18% for attention deficit. None of the other classroom factors account for more than 10% of the variance and this is for classroom attendance. The low R^2 values show that this is a weak model on which to base the conclusion.

Third, the nutritional variable was dichotomous and the use of a dichotomous variable is a questionable procedure. The authors in a footnote quote Kim and Mueller who consider that a dichotomous variable may be used "as a means of finding a clustering of variables". This does not extend the use of multiple regression analyses for the purpose of examining causal factors.

Finally, the conclusion ignores the possibility that the impairments of the malnourished children at follow-up may have been caused in part, or in some cases wholly, by the environmental histories of the children subsequent to malnutrition.

Both the Jamaican and Barbados studies laboured under the difficulty of not having a good general conceptual basis for studying child development or well developed measures that describe significant experiences in the history of a child. In the Barbados study the only environment considered was the family. This may be appropriate for infants, but if the histories of children up to age 11 are to be accounted for there are other microenvironments that may influence children; e.g., the neighbourhood, the school, peer relationships. Perhaps the most useful general conceptualization of child development that considers the environment is given by Bronfenbrenner (2) in *The Ecology of Child Development*. My Fig. 1 is a summary of his conceptual schema. Given the early stages in research into the environmental histories of children, it is premature with the rather crude measures and analyses that have been used in malnutrition research to claim that malnutrition plays an important causative role in later intellectual and social impairment.

1. Galler, J. (ed.) (1984). *In* "Nutrition and Behaviour", Chap. 3, p. 101, Plenum Press, New York.
2. Bronfenbrenner, U. (1980). "The Ecology of Child Development". Harvard University Press, Cambridge, MA.

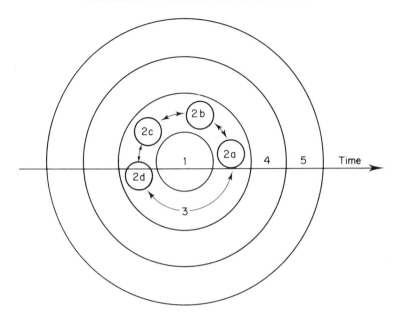

Fig. 1. Bronfenbrenner's schema of the ecology of human development with definitions of the components of the schema. From (2).

(1) The developing human being.

(2)[a] "A *microsystem* is a pattern of activities, roles, and interpersonal relations experienced by the developing person in a given setting[b] (a,b,c, etc.) with particular physical and material characteristics." (p.22).

(3)[a] "A *mesosystem* comprises the interrelations among two or more settings in which the developing person actively participates (such as for a child, the relations among home, school, and neighborhood peer group; for an adult, among family, work and social life)." (p.25).

(4)[c] "An *exosystem* refers to one or more settings that do not involve the developing person as a participant, but in which events occur that affect, or are affected by, what happens in the setting containing the developing person." (p.25).

(5)[c] "The *macrosystem* refers to consistencies, in the form and content of lower-order systems (micro-, meso- and exo) that exist or could exist, at the level of the subculture or the culture as a whole, along with any belief systems or ideology underlying such consistencies." (p.26).

[a] Direct Interaction. [b] A setting is a place where people can readily engage in face-to-face interaction, e.g. home, playground, school. (p.22). [c] Indirect Interaction.

D. A. Levitsky and Barbara J. Strupp: Galler has given us a review of the most controversial question in the entire malnutrition/behaviour literature: does early malnutrition have a long-term effect on cognitive functioning *independently* of the role of environment? Although Galler hedges her answer ("The role of the environment has still to be finally assessed."), it is clear from her paper, as well as from her many important contributions to the literature, that she firmly believes that it does.

Accepting such an answer represents one of two alternative hypotheses concerning the nature of the effect of early malnutrition on cognitive development. We shall call these two positions, the "Hardware" and the "Software" hypotheses. The Hardware hypothesis, which Galler maintains, holds that malnutrition occurring during critical times in early development causes irreversible damage to those brain structures (Hardware) that are responsible for optimal cognitive functioning. Alternatively, the Software hypothesis rejects the brain damage position and maintains that during the period of malnutrition the organism may be "distracted" from learning those aspects of its environment that are important for optimal cognitive functioning later in life. The Software position places a far greater role on the environment as a major determinate of any long-term effect of malnutrition on cognition than does the Hardware hypothesis.

Galler uses two arguments in her paper to convince us of the Hardware hypothesis. Her first argument is based upon the observation that many studies have found that children exposed to malnutrition display long-term alterations in some aspects of cognitive functioning. Of this fact, there is no debate. Then, Galler proceeds to explain those studies that have not found cognitive impairments in children who have been malnourished, not because of a lack of food to eat, but rather because of problems related to an organic illness.

Such evidence would be damaging to the Hardware hypothesis for two reasons. First, brain growth in these children would be expected to be inhibited to a similar degree as children who were malnourished because of lack of food; the Hardware would be expected to be damaged. And second, the poor environmental conditions that usually cohabitate with malnutrition are absent in these studies, suggesting that the cause of the cognitive deficits in children suffering from malnutrition is more directly related to the poor environmental conditions than the brain growth inhibition. Galler's rebuttal to such evidence is that "There are too few studies, based on small sample sizes, and for the most part, there are major limitations in the selection of control groups".

But can enough of these kinds of studies be done, or the sample sizes be sufficiently large, or the control groups be adequately matched to ever prove the null hypothesis that malnutrition does not cause cognitive impairment? The answer is no, not because of the veracity of the Hardware hypothesis, but rather because the nature of the scientific method does not allow the proof of the null hypothesis, only its disproof. Therefore, although Galler's rebuttal must be accepted as logically true, the force of such an argument is weak; it is impossible to ever prove that malnutrition *does not* cause cognitive impairment.

The other argument Galler raises in defence of the Hardware hypothesis is based on her own data. Utilizing a relatively unique natural situation where the population is homogeneous and non-mobile, yet sufficiently heterogenous that malnutrition does occur, Galler and her colleagues were able to study children with a history of early malnutrition through their early school years. Although there were many important findings from this study, the most pertinent for this discussion is that children with a history of malnutrition displayed significantly lower IQ scores than their controls, *independently* of the effect of environment from which they were raised. This is a very significant finding, for if true, it is the best evidence available for the Hardware hypothesis.

There are some worrying aspects about this finding, however, that might severely limit the ability to generalize these findings, a concern that is also shared by Galler. The most obvious of these concerns is the disparity in findings between the Galler study and those of the Jamaican studies (her refs 35, 47–50). The design of the two studies was very similar. Yet, the Jamaican studies showed an overwhelming effect of environment on almost all behavioural and cognitive measures, similar to that found by most developmental studies that have measured environmental factors and children's cognitive performance. But as Table 1 indicates, the Barbados study shows almost no effect of environment on Full Scale IQ or Verbal IQ. Only on the Performance IQ measurement did environment sneak through as a significant factor.

Galler explains this discrepancy in findings by arguing that the environments were considerably more homogeneous in Barbardos than in Jamaica. This could very well be true. As any student of experimental design knows, the ability to detect a significant correlation depends, in part, upon the range of scores used in the analysis. It would be difficult to detect an effect of environment if the range of values for the environmental factors was small.

However, an alternative explanation is that the particular measures Galler used to estimate the environment of the children in Barbados were not sufficiently sensitive to detect real differences in environmental conditions between the Index children and the Comparison children that may have actually existed. Since Galler used Nutrition and Environment as the two major independent variables in her statistical models, if the measures of Environment proved to be poor indicators of reality, then all the residual effects in the children's scores would be attributed to Nutrition. The burden of proof of the contention that malnutrition causes decrements in cognitive functioning independent of environment lies with the demonstration that the indicators of environmental conditions used in the statistical analysis of the IQ data were, indeed, sensitive and accurate measures of reality.

One final point deserves mention. Galler fails to mention the findings of the Dutch Famine study (1) in which no indication of any cognitive impairment was evident in young adults subjected to a brief period of perinatal malnutrition. This is a very important study, and although it contains some methodological limitations, it should be included in a discussion concerning the long-term effects of early malnutrition on cognition.

1. Stein, Z., Susser, M., Saenger, G. and Marolla, F. (1975). "Famine and Human Development". Oxford University Press, London.

J. Dobbing: I have two general comments on Levitsky's Commentary on Galler's paper, both of them somewhat peripheral to its main theme, but, I think, important nonetheless. The first is a strong condemnation of the use of the term "damage" when referring to the effects of early undernutrition on the brain. It must be clearly understood that "damage" in this context has a very precise connotation in neuropathology, and in this sense has never been part of the neuropathology of nutritional growth restriction. Damage means that some brain tissue has been destroyed, that like all destruction of brain tissue it cannot ever be replaced, and in the field of paediatric neuropathology it implies more or less severe malfunction (mental retardation in the true sense) which, like the lesion, is permanent. Early nutritional deprivation *has never been shown to result in brain damage.* The most malnutrition does to the "Hardware" is to make deficits and distortions in it by altering its development. Nothing is destroyed. The misuse of the word in this context is serious, not only for doctrinaire, semantic reasons: it strikes at the heart of all we know of the capacity of most people to compensate functionally for a poor nutritional babyhood. Secondly it is unkind to parents and misleading to politicians and those who fund research, for all of whom "brain damage" means the same as it does to neuropathologists: irrecoverable doom. Please will Levitsky (and for that matter Richardson) resolve not to use the expression ever again in this context?

Secondly, can we please not follow Levitsky in placing the Dutch famine study so high on the list of literature important to our subject? The failure of the Dutch army authorities (no more sophisticated in the 1960s than any other military organization when assessing fine grain differences in intellectual achievement) to detect any deleterious effect of a famine lasting only a period of months, often not even during much of the brain growth spurt, and never involving more than one third of its duration, is without any serious impact on our subject. All they would have detected by these methods would have been quite serious mental retardation of a kind that even the army would not find acceptable for service, and which none of us would responsibly suggest to be a consequence of early malnutrition. The Dutch famine study was excellent, its conclusions about maternal nutrition and fetal growth seminal, its opportunism brilliant, but it should not be raised to the stature of "a very important study" for our present subject.

D. E. Barrett: I personally think Galler is correct in concluding, without equivocation, that severe malnutrition early in life is one important environmental factor which has long-term, adverse effects on intellectual development. Second, her suggestion of a role of disturbances in the mother–child relationship as a mediator of the effects of early malnutrition on later behaviour is useful. She reminds us that while such disruptions are a likely mediator of identified relationships between early undernutrition and later behaviour impairment, such influences may also mediate the adverse behavioural effects of other types of risks to the organism. She also shows that the effects of early and severe malnutrition in the child on the behaviour of the care-giver toward the child are not always the same. Thus, while early and severe malnutrition is likely to affect the mother–child relationship, the specific effects on the mother's behaviour, for example, whether she becomes overprotective or neglecting, may depend on certain social variables. Third, I think Galler is correct in her insistence on the need for repeated measurements of environmental variables if one is to understand the role of those variables, independent of or in interaction with nutritional variables, in the prediction of later behaviour outcomes.

I do not think that the distinction Galler has drawn between retrospective and longitudinal studies is a useful one; in fact I think it leads to some confusion.

Galler is attempting to distinguish studies on the basis of how the samples were obtained. The studies Galler describes as "retrospective" are those generally referred to as "cross-sectional" (a term Galler also uses). In these studies, subjects are selected from a population without regard for standing on the independent or dependent variables of interest. Independent and dependent variables are then related (using, for example, a correlation approach) across subjects. Fleiss (1,2) calls this type of approach "method I sampling." Again, this type of study is distinguished from other types of studies in that subjects are not chosen for the study because of their standing on the independent variable ("method II sampling") or dependent variable ("method II sampling").

Once the data have been obtained, they can be analysed using a retrospective or prospective analysis (or a correlational analysis which is neither retrospective nor prospective). For example, in the Cravioto *et al.* (3) study, the data analysis is prospective: from presumed antecedent to presumed consequent variable. Specifically, children in a "good nutritional history" group (i.e. tallest children) are compared with children in a "poor nutritional history" group (shortest children) on the behavioural variables. If the authors had, instead, identified the children who had performed best on the intersensory tasks (e.g. scored in the highest quartile) and those that had performed most poorly and then computed the odds ratios for likelihood of falling in the first as opposed to the fourth height quartiles, this would be a retrospective analysis; from presumed consequent to presumed antecedent.

Galler characterizes studies in this group as involving classifications of nutritional history based on inference, questioning or review of records, but this is not an essential feature of method I studies.

The studies Galler describes as longitudinal are those Fleiss calls method II, prospective. Subjects are identified who have a certain standing or status on an independent variable of interest. A second group is identified that differs on the independent variable. The groups are compared on selected dependent variables. (More than two groups can be compared.)

All of the studies which Galler describes as longitudinal fit the above definition. However, studies at only two points in time which she describes as longitudinal are longitudinal in the sense that the term is usually defined. For example, Champakam *et al.* (4) and Klein *et al.* (5) examined subjects at only one outcome time (i.e. one occasion per subject).

Further, I disagree with Galler's statement that the studies which she describes as longitudinal "have advantages over retrospective studies in that they allow the evaluation of causal relationships between an earlier event and later outcome". As non-experimental comparison studies, they are subject to many of the threats to internal validity (6,7) that method I studies are subject to. Logical inferences about causal effects can be made without experimentation if explicit causal models are empirically tested, but this can be accomplished with data from both method I and method II studies.

1. Fleiss, J. L. (1973). "Statistical Methods for Rates and Proportions". John Wiley, New York.
2. Fleiss, J. L. (1981). "Statistical Methods for Rates and Proportions" 2nd edn. John Wiley, New York.
3. Cravioto, J., DeLicardie, E. R. and Birch, H. G. (1966). Nutrition, growth and neurointegrative development: an experimental and ecologic study. *Pediat.* **38**, 319–372.
4. Champakam, S., Srikantia, S. and Gopalan, C. (1968). Kwashiorkor and mental development. *Am. J. Clin. Nutr.* **21**, 844–852.
5. Klein, P. S., Forbes, G. B. and Nader, P. R. (1975). Effects of starvation in infancy (pyloric stenosis) on subsequent learning abilities. *J. Pediat.* **87**, 8–15.
6. Cook, T. D. and Campbell, D. T. (1979). "Quasi-experimentation: Design and Analysis for Field Settings." Rand-McNally, Chicago.
7. Barrett, D. E. (1984). Methodological requirements for conceptually valid research studies on the behavioral effects of malnutrition. *In* "Nutrition and Behavior" (J. R. Galler, ed.) pp. 9–36. Plenum Press, New York.

K. S. Bedi: Once again the conclusions drawn in this paper are the same: the environment in which a child is reared probably affects the later behavioural development; isolation of the environmental factors from the nutritional ones is not easy.

In my previous commentary on Grantham-McGregor's paper I stated that "humans simply do not make good experimental material for such studies", because of the difficulties of defining, let alone isolating, all the various environmental factors which could be involved. Galler's paper reinforces this. She outlines the possible factors she has considered in her research work, and I have counted 20 or so factors she has listed. Some of these have subgroups, some are obviously interrelated and some probably counterbalance others in unknown ways. How can one possibly sort out this mess and ascribe "figures" to them?

I. Hurwitz: This presentation begins with a review of the relative advantages and disadvantages of studies of malnutrition effects, utilizing both retrospective and longitudinal designs. The benefits and flaws of both approaches have been well documented in other reports, though Galler does make the point that longitudinal studies have for the most part been most informative with respect to adverse outcomes, particularly with regard to intellectual deficit. That intellectual deficit is most often reported, is not necessarily because of the special vulnerability of intelligence to the effects of malnutrition, but rather is more likely due to the accessibility of measuring devices of this construct to researchers. Galler points out the more recent research efforts in this field of malnutrition have broadened the range of dependent variables studied to include school performances and social emotional behaviours as well as intelligence, particularly in more recent investigations. One might comment at this point, however, that in reference to the South African study, the value of the Harris–Goodenough, a drawing task of the human figure, is somewhat questionable as an indicator of "emotional immaturity". The extensive array of reports included in Galler's paper does unquestionably point to IQ measures as reflecting the damaging consequences of various sorts of malnutrition and undernutrition in countries throughout the developing world, yet the dubious nature and ambiguities that surround the question of what constitutes "intelligence" continue to plague researchers in their effort to understand what it mediates as well as of what it is constituted, in terms of relevant underlying processes and functions. When researchers "close in" on the concept through the study of such activities as intersensory integration, problem solving, school performance, etc., then perhaps there results a closer grasp of what Barrett has referred to as measurable variables which lend themselves to operational definitions and quantification. However, these outcome considerations, given the title of Galler's paper, particularly the use of the term "interaction" in the context of nutrition and environment, demand a somewhat different focus in this commentary. Few would argue nowadays that the environmental circumstances in which children are raised, where nutritional deficits exist, represent a major determinant in the eventual outcomes observed. Yet Galler acknowledges that this issue may not be as self-evident to investigators as it appears when she states ". . . malnourished children most often come from the lowest socioeconomic classes of the population. When impaired intellectual performance is documented in these children, there has been a tendency to oversimplify this relationship and to attribute behavioural deficits primarily to nutritional factors without taking adequate account of environmental factors or to environmental factors alone". There follows then an account of a wide array of these environmental variables and a number of studies which have explored their role in both prospective (Cravioto and DeLicardie) and retrospective investigations (Grantham-MacGregor). What is most interesting in Galler's report is her review of studies which now appear to assign significance to the quality and nature of the mother–child interactions, influences which must be regarded as having vital significance on a par with economic, social and demographic factors. Cultural attitudes and practices, temperament of child and mother, nutritional values, etc., i.e. those microenvironmental variables which directly impact on the child and family, may prove to be the most significant issues to consider in any future research efforts, and by implication as well as in recent fact, provide us with the basis for the most important areas of intervention which may be supplied along with essential nutritional supplementation programmes.

Galler provides us with a list of environmental factors which indeed appear relevant and plausible, though they lack theoretical consistency in an integrative sense. Nonetheless, their means of interaction is never clearly elucidated other than to suggest that factor analytic methods may condense seemingly divergent variables into conceptually useful categories.

It still remains for multivariate methods and still more sophisticated statistical procedures such as discriminant function analysis to clarify further the hierarchic contribution of non-nutritional environmental factors in conjunction with malnutrition in understanding the complex issues surrounding behavioural outcomes.

S. Richardson: Hurwitz's statement that various sorts of malnutrition and undernutrition *unquestionably* have damaging consequences was felt by many of us to be too general a conclusion to make from the research evidence in human studies. Different forms of malnutrition and undernutrition may have different effects in different social contexts and the relative effects of the *direct* consequences are far from being understood in each case.

Sally Grantham-McGregor: I cannot agree with Hurwitz that the "array of reports included in Galler's paper do *unquestionably* point to IQ measures as reflecting the damaging consequences of various sorts of malnutrition and undernutrition in countries throughout the developing world". Galler mostly reviewed studies involving severe malnutrition. The weight of evidence from these studies suggests that in children returning to poor environments *marasmus* has a detrimental effect on mental development, at least up to adolescence.

Linda S. Crnic: The body of literature on the effects of malnutrition caused by conditions such as pyloric stenosis and cystic fibrosis is of immense theoretical and practical importance. Therefore I must protest against Galler's dismissal of this literature on the basis that it is scant and inconclusive. While I would not argue with the desirability for more data, the concordance amongst the studies on this topic is striking in view of the general lack of agreement in the field. I must also disagree with the assessment that these sorts of studies can isolate the effects of environment from nutrition. While children from privileged environments who suffer from malnutrition produced by these disorders are not reared in the adverse environment associated with starvation resulting from poverty, they are *not* growing up in a normal environment. They have spent substantial time in the stressful and deprived environment of the hospital. Their illness often has strained family finances. The birth and care of a child with serious illness is often a stimulus for family discord and divorce (1). Because these children are stunted, and therefore look younger than their age, it is likely that expectations for their performance are lowered and they are treated as if they were younger. In addition, there is a tendency to infantalize children because of their illness and consequent extra need for care (2).

On the other hand, one might well postulate beneficial effects of the increased attention an ill child is likely to receive. In sum, while it is difficult to assess whether the environmental alterations would be helpful or harmful to the child, it is clear that the environment is not normal. An additional consideration is that the malnutrition in these cases is likely to be circumscribed in severity and duration. Thus, while these studies are of extreme importance, they must be carefully interpreted because their ability to separate environmental from nutritional effects is in fact limited.

One very important contribution of Galler's studies has been to point out to us that environment, as well as malnutrition can have different effects on different areas of function. In addition, she postulates that the relationship between nutrition and environment might be a function of the quality of the environment: fewer effects of environment were seen in her studies of Barbadian children growing up in a relatively "enriched" environment whereas others have found more evidence for environmental effects in children from other, more "impoverished" environments. As is usual in science, it is valuable to refine general concepts like "effects of environment on behaviour" to accommodate specific concerns with the effects of particular aspects of the environment on specific classes of behaviour. In this context it is important to consider that malnourished children in industrialized societies come from unstable homes, as Galler notes, and further that their malnutrition is often part of a picture of abuse and neglect. Thus, we must anticipate an especially potent interaction between the environment of abuse and the effects of malnutrition upon the social and emotional development of these children.

1. Prugh, D. G. and Eckhardt, L. O. (1980). Children's reaction to illness, hospitalization and surgery. *In* "Comprehensive Textbook of Psychiatry" (H. I. Kaplan, A. M. Freedman and B. J. Sadock, eds) Vol. III. Williams and Wilkins, Baltimore, MD.
2. Finch, S. M. (1980). Psychological factors affecting physical conditions. *In* "Comprehensive Textbook of Psychiatry" (H. I. Kaplan, A. M. Freedman and B. J. Sadock, eds) Vol. III, pp. 2505–2513. Williams and Wilkins, Baltimore, MD.

Sally Grantham-McGregor: Galler reports her findings from Barbados. This is another study with a similar design to those reviewed in the first part of the chapter, and has similar findings. The index children had lower scores on tests of IQ and school achievement than the control children. She reports that both the environment and a previous history of malnutrition explain some of the variance in IQ. This has been found many times before.

As Galler rightly says, it is impossible to measure all factors in the environment. I am not sure that it is useful to stress that a past history of malnutrition is more important than the current environment, or vice versa. This will depend on what is measured in the environment and how sensitive the instruments were in detecting differences. The fact that malnutrition had a greater effect on the mental development in this study than in the Jamaican study carried out by Richardson *et al.* cannot be substantiated by the analysis, because different environmental factors were measured differently. It may be that her instruments were not as sensitive as those used in the Jamaican study. What is important is that *both studies* found that both the environment and a history of malnutrition contributed to the variance in IQ.

One of the strengths of the Barbados study which is not emphasized is that there were records of the nutritional status of the control children in early childhood and this is often not the case. The fact that they were not undernourished as well may partly explain the fairly large difference between the groups.

I have problems with Galler's definition of *marasmus*. This is usually restricted to children with weight below 60% of expected value. It is very confusing when she uses "florid marasmus" to describe her samples in her first paper where she also states the children were below 75% of expected weight for age. When she refers to "unpublished data" which shows no difference in IQ between children who suffered from kwashiorkor and marasmus it would be nice to know what is meant by "marasmus".

Longitudinal observational studies do not allow "evaluation of causal relationships" as suggested by Galler. It is therefore *not possible to prove cause* from the study design used in the Barbados study.

However, I think it is reasonable to attribute a causal relationship between marasmus and poor mental development in poor environments when one considers the whole weight of evidence of all the studies reviewed by Galler. This conclusion was also reached by Pollitt and Thomson (1).

A further point of interest is that Galler reports that the socioeconomic status of the malnourished Barbados group was better than that usually found in formerly malnourished children. It has been suggested in the past, especially when referring to the studies from developing countries, that the effects of malnutrition are less in these circumstances. However, we have very little real evidence for this statement.

It is also interesting that in her analysis, no interaction was found between environment and malnutrition. This is another point which is often accepted, again without evidence.

1. Pollitt, E. and Thomson, C. (1977). Protein–calorie malnutrition and behaviour: a review from psychology. *In* "Nutrition and the Brain" (R. J. Wurtman and J. J. Wurtman, eds) Vol. 2, pp. 261–306. Raven Press, New York.

Studies on Poverty, Human Growth and Development: The Cali Experience

LEONARDO SINISTERRA

Fundación de Investigaciones de Ecologia Humana, Apartado Aéreo 7308, Cali, Colombia

Introduction

It is now well accepted that the level of growth and development attained by the children of a community is the best index of the general level of cultural and economic development of the community and of the country as a whole. Developed countries have well developed citizens.

For historical reasons which are not difficult to understand, the tropical and subtropical areas of the world have secularly shown restricted social, economic, scientific, and human growth and development. It is now possible to discern the relationship between physical and human development. We know that humans and their environment interact and that, in the final analysis, one is partly a cause and at the same time a consequence of the other.

This evidence of the close relationship between the living human being and his environment — social, physical and emotional — prompted the group of medical researchers, nutritionists and educational experts in Cali (Colombia), to enter the field of human growth and development. The group had a clear objective of producing information for the sake of science, but was also basically moved by the urgent ethical need to do something for the chronic

Early Nutrition and Later Achievement
ISBN: 0-12-218855-1

and alarming human inequalities which were causing disastrous morbidity, mortality, and other medical problems amongst the poorer children of those Cali communities which were emerging as a consequence of the massive rural–urban migration typical of the developing world in the 1960s and '70s.

The task has been a difficult one, with many frustrations and almost as many satisfactions, and has lasted much longer than initially expected. Today, when we see that two and a half decades have elapsed and that there is still much to do and learn, we feel more than ever that this must be our duty, and that if we were given the chance to start again, we would follow the same course.

The Socioeconomic Context

Population distribution, though relatively stable for generations, has precipitously changed in the last 30 years. Rural inhabitants have massively migrated to the cities, looking for better living conditions, jobs, health, education and the other advantages of modern urban life. Latin American populations have been particularly prone to the tendency of urbanization. The Population Reference Bureau (1) reports that: "the total population of the continent which was close to 180 million people in 1950 (about 80 million in urban areas and 100 in rural sectors) will reach 600 million by the year 2000 (480 million in urban and 120 in rural sectors)". Thus urban areas in 50 years time could see their population increase from 80 to 480 million. This process has been going on for the last 30 years and in 1986 we have approximately 300 million inhabitants in the cities and 110 in rural areas (Fig. 1).

Colombia has been no exception. The 1951 Colombian census showed a total population of 11·5 million; the 1985 census 26·5 million. With a similar urban–rural distribution, the Colombian urban population was 4·5 million in 1951 and 18·5 million in 1985 (Fig. 2).

Under these conditions cities are overcrowded and public services (water supply, electricity, sewage systems) are insufficient to meet the population's needs; education and health services are scant and of low quality; other aspects of social intercourse such as employment and recreation are also limited. The "poverty belts" surrounding the large capitals and the intermediate cities of countries in Latin America, from Mexico to Argentina, are appalling. The scene is practically the same in all 20 countries, whether the people speak French, as in Port au Prince; or Portuguese, as in the *favelas* of Rio de Janiero; or Spanish, as in the Chilean Cayampa, the "young towns" of Lima, the slums of Bogota, Cali, or Caracas, or the astonishing 17 million of Mexico City.

This phenomenon of overcrowding with different causes from one country to another, but having similar consequences in all, is the dominant sociological problem of the Latin American continent.

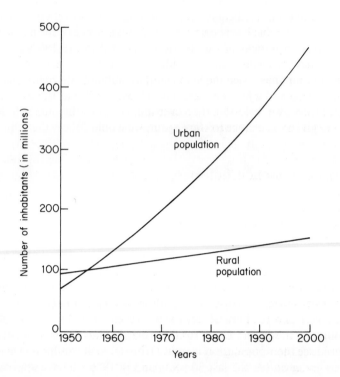

Fig. 1. Latin American population growth: urban and rural increment 1950–2000. From (1).

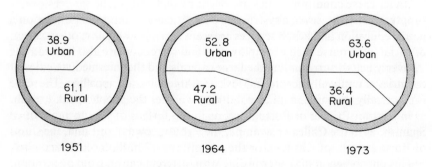

Fig. 2. Colombia: percentage of urban and rural populations, 1978. Source: Colombian Institute of Statistics (DANE).

Crowding, unemployment, promiscuity and a chronic feeling of hopelessness and defeat dominate human life in the slums of squatter towns. The vulnerable groups in these settlements are those under physiological stress, for example pregnant women, lactating mothers, preschool children and adolescents. Women, frequently mothers of young children, are forced to join the labour force, leaving their children unprotected and unattended. Reduced incomes imply poor diets. The contaminated environment is a permanent threat to their health; and finally malnutrition and infection join forces synergistically to the common detriment.

The consequences are easy to foresee. Repeated visits to Health Centres or hospitals are part of everyday life; relapses are just as frequent since treatments given are no more than palliative or symptomatic. The tragic thing for the health professions is that the consequences of poverty and malnutrition are frequently clinical, but their causes are not. Another important effect of poverty is the psychological and emotional damage caused to children. They become unfriendly, unsociable and aggressive. At age 7 when they first go to school, they fail, which is not surprising. As might be expected, the migration of large population groups from the relatively grey, but easy life in the rural areas, to the colourful but poverty-stricken life in the cities, has made a great impact on the minds and programmes of medical educators, researchers and practitioners.

The poverty in which most immigrant families live affects all aspects of the slum dweller's life. Housing facilities are very poor and poor hygiene is always present. Poor nutrition is inevitable and this affects the most vulnerable groups. Body defences weaken and infections are frequent; the crowded conditions favour communicable disease and the synergistic forces of malnutrition and infection contribute to the deterioration of the community's health.

The increasing number of children hospitalized and dying has moved the medical authorities to pay more attention to the problem. Unfortunately, it has taken a long time for other professionals and governments to initiate programmes seeking to solve it. In the author's own Department of Nutrition a mixture has been developed to help alleviate hunger amongst the children. After several trials, this became a mixture of soya beans and rice containing 19% protein enriched with vitamins and minerals. The product, Colombiharina (2), was well accepted by both adults and children. Currently over 1200 tons are produced annually and sold at a price of US $0·5 per kg, about 15% of the price of the same amount of powdered milk. A nutritional recovery ward was also organized in the Department of Nutrition and operated jointly with the Department of Pediatrics in the University Hospital. Results from those initial years, mostly in relation to intestinal malabsorption, the role of folic acid and haematological responses, are found in several publications (3).

Our experience with the recovery of malnourished children in a hospital was highly educational. After two years more than 100 children had been treated, yet nearly 70% of them had been readmitted for a relapse in their condition. This experience led us to move out of the hospital to a Health Centre in the heart of the community where most of the hospital children came from. Here we organized a Nutrition, *Education* and Recovery Unit. Colombiharina was our main tool. Through the child we established immediate contact with the family and during the next four years we learned a great deal about the real conditions of life. Two lines were pursued: the promotion of Colombiharina and other vegetable mixtures to alleviate hunger and the recognition that solving the nutritional problem alone was not enough. Even after children had physically recovered it was relatively easy to see that they suffered emotional, psychological and social retardation. Children of 5 and 6 years behaved like toddlers of 2 or 3. Colombiharina repeatedly proved to be excellent for physical recuperation, but useless in face of the mental impact of malnutrition and chronic deprivation.

In the course of our field work we came to know the families of the children we treated very well. In this way we found that the children were as retarded as their parents. Not surprisingly the child had a mental stature which matched his family and community environment. This observation was critically important for our future work.

It is not the function of scientists to change the economic and political structure of a society, but it is our responsibility to understand its inequalities and limitations because it is within this context that we must exercise our knowledge. We cannot close our eyes to the surrounding reality and limit our work to the "simulated" conditions of the laboratory or even of the hospital. Medical and para-medical groups must discover strategies for survival under real conditions, and try to reduce to a minimum the physical and psychological impact of malnutrition, and this will mean accepting social restrictions.

Our Early Childhood Intervention Research Programmes

Experience in our Health Centre's Unit of Nutrition, Education and Recuperation led us to organize facilities for the systematic study and evaluation of the effects of multiple deprivations on human health, and particularly on the behaviour of underprivileged children. Following our interest in the impact of deprivation on behavioural development, our initial focus was on the identification of specific aspects of psychological development which are negatively affected by poor health and nutritional deficits, as well as by other environmental deprivations. A wide variety of psychological measures were used to specify those characteristics most clearly retarded by chronic poor health and deficient nutrition.

The social–affective or social–emotional development of young children is particularly hard to measure. Ironically it is these characteristics of malnourished children that are so obvious to those of us who have worked with them daily. We constantly observed characteristics such as apathy, sadness, and fearfulness. These changed dramatically with changed life circumstances, better diet, and better health. It was difficult, however, to design a series of situation-specific observation scales that could move us from our purely clinical observations to a level where we could quantify the variables and show that what we observed was not just misperception due to a desire to see such behavioural manifestations. To accomplish this we trained a group of behavioural observation specialist helpers to gather reliable information using several different scales.

Our professional group also became interested in further understanding two areas which were critical for the development of applicable and relevant knowledge. Within the first area we then attempted to identify the types of intervention necessary to overcome the various damaging effects of early malnutrition. This involved direct and sustained nutritional supplementation, behavioural stimulation, and medical treatment. The question was whether powerful behavioural stimulation and nutritional supplementation could overcome the retardation of these children. If it could be overcome, up to what age and for which psychological functions?

The second area was the investigation of the relationship between specific deficits (and their amelioration) and the actual academic and social success of these children once they were in school.

We concluded that children must develop a wide range of socially effective behaviours by the time they reach school age if they are to become useful members of societies and participate fully in culturally valued aspects of contemporary urban life. Unfortunately little was known at that time about important, identifiable, and changeable components of the psychological ability of young children. It could have been that poor development of affective, attentional, social, and other *non-cognitive* psychological characteristics were the most serious result of poor nutrition and environmental deprivation.

In practical terms at that time we reached the conclusion that a greater variety of behavioural measurement was needed to study the effects of nutrional deficits and supplementation, because it might be that an expanded range of behavioural descriptions, relevant to an individual's preparation for productive social roles, could provide a clearer description of the deficits produced by multiple deprivations. These findings might help us identify the types of interventions necessary to overcome the various damaging effects of early malnutrition. Therefore our initial model of intervention should involve direct and sustained nutritional supplementation, behavioural stimulation, and medical care.

In summary, the three main measurement objectives in this initial stage of our work, were: (a) identifying the specific aspects of psychological development retarded by nutritional, health, and other environmental deficits; (b) identifying which of the retardations were modifiable through various means; and (c) identifying the relevance of the modifiable or non-modifiable behaviour for future life.

The complete list of the proposed behavioural measurements is described in *Nutrition, Development and Social Behaviour* (4). The list includes measures of success in school as well as in the social–affective area.

We thus used all these tests and scales to measure human development in this research area, keeping always in mind the need to expand them to include reliable assessment of social–affective responses, as well as more clearly articulated cognitive and intellectual skill development. Furthermore, we stressed the need to emphasize the relevance of the variable studied to the child's success or failure in life, in terms of the child as a human resource and as a satisfaction-seeking organism.

General Methodological Problems and Decisions Taken

The very complex interrelationships among health, nutrition, and family factors in the psychological development of young children can only be studied by adopting an intervention model as the primary research mechanism. The quasiexperimental model (5) we finally adopted was based on nutritional, medical, and behavioural intervention whose purpose was to assess direct treatment effects.

For the operation of our programmes we selected areas of the city composed primarily of very low income families. A preliminary survey was made of the area to obtain a count of all children living there who were within the birth-dates specified by our experimental design, and to verify that living conditions indicated a very low economic level.

This general preparatory methodology yielded groups in the experiments, that were (a) virtually equivalent to each other, and (b) represented the larger community in an unbiased way. We selected children coming from families in which the average income per person per month was about US $5·00, with no additional sources of food or other goods. They had a mean weight and length below the third percentile of the Boston norms, an average of more than ten clinical signs of malnutrition (6), and five to six dental caries. We found TB exposure in 10% and histories of chronic diarrhoea and vomiting in over 50%. Nearly 75% had an abnormally high parasite count and 15%

had extensive skin infections. All were evaluated in medical terms as having poor health.

Specific Intervention Studies: Designs and Sample Results

In all of our intervention studies (two pilot studies and one longitudinal study) we used the same basic experimental design with the following types of major treatments:

Type A
                             behavioural stimulation
Test . . . .   plus   . . . . retest
                        nutritional and health care
Type B
Test . . . . nutritional and health care . . . . retest
Type C
Test . . . . no treatment . . . . retest

This experimental design missed a group which would have made a neat two-by-two factorial design; that is, a group receiving behavioural stimulation but not nutritional and health care. For children who were receiving limited amounts of food at home, and who were nutritionally losing ground every month, such treatment would have contributed to their increasingly hazardous undernutrition in the face of the added risk of cross-infection in the group. Our studies never included such controls. Our studies did assess the relative benefits of behavioural intervention plus nutritional treatment compared to those receiving the nutritional treatment alone.

Within each of the major types of treatment variables we further subdivided each study in different ways. This design enabled the use of the analysis of variance and provided a wealth of information regarding interactions among the major treatments and the minor variations within them.

The first pilot study

The first short-term multifactorial experiment included the following groups (4):

Type A CS: Cognitive stimulation plus nutritional and health care
        PS: Physical stimulation plus nutritional and health care
Type B LS: Low stimulation (free play) plus nutritional and health care
Type C CO: Control, no treatment, siblings of treated children

In this study, all children were from low-income families and presented a clinical and anthropometric picture of having endured chronic undernutrition.

Groups were similar in mean age and nutritional status indicators. The treatment of the three participating groups lasted four months. At the end of the experiment, all three groups had similar rates of nutritional physical recovery.

The cognitive stimulation (CS) group received a four-month programme of highly concentrated verbal activity, and experience in object and concept classification and generalization, while the physical stimulation (PS) group was simply kept at a high peak of daily motor activity during the same four-month period. The low stimulation (LS) group was kept at the Health Centre with a caretaker and several types of toys and games to play, but was not directed to behave in any special way except for feeding and hygiene.

Summary findings of this first pilot study include:

(1) The LS group did not show improvement in any of the measures used in the study as a result of receiving a good diet for four months, even though their measures of health and nutritional status increased more rapidly than those of controls. In cognitive development (Knox Cubes, Fig. 3) as well as in the use of letters (reading), this group seemed to be developing during the four-month period at a rate no better than that of untreated controls. This was also found to be true in the second Pilot Study. Improved nutrition then seems only to ameliorate physical growth and health, with no perceptible psychological repercussion.

(2) The performance on the Knox Cubes seemed resistant to treatment with the method used in this study; treated groups responded no better than controls. This result, coupled with data from the Memory for Sentences test, very close to zero, suggested to us that the undernourished child's retardation of short-term memory is especially resistant to treatment, whether behavioural and/or nutritional.

(3) The highly verbal treatment of the CS group did not yield gains superior to those found in the physically very active PS group. The same results were found among all "basic" cognitive measures. These results suggested that the different types of behavioural treatment provided yielded equal experience in readiness to learn verbal relationships, and this was higher than in non-behaviourally treated children (LS).

(4) Behavioural stimulation (physical and cognitive) improved basic intellectual capabilities to a moderate degree, while dramatically improving specific task achievement. However, the goal was far from realized, as some of the measures remained unaltered with treatment.

The second pilot study

Our second pilot study lasted five months, rather than four. The behavioural treatment was the same for all children; this time we did not have a

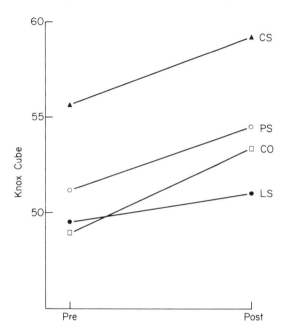

Fig. 3. Knox Cubes test score changes over the four-month period of the first pilot study. Test scores are standard scores (mean = 50, SD = 10) based on norms for children from subject *barrio* (CS = cognitive stimulation plus nutritional and health care; PS = physical stimulation plus nutritional and health care; LS = low stimulation, free play, plus nutritional and health care; CO = control, no treatment, siblings of treated children). From (4).

physical stimulation group. The sequence of stimulation was better established, the teachers more experienced, and the activities more varied. This time two secondary variables were more systematically considered: nutritional level at the start of the programme, and "spill-over" effects to undernourished siblings of the treated children.

For this second study, we included, in the cognitive stimulation programme, a group of nutritionally normal children from the same poor neighbourhoods and mixed them with the malnourished group. In order to avoid what might have been negative effects suffered by the low stimulation (LS) children in the first study, we decided to treat the group receiving only food and health care by delivering their food at their homes and bringing the children to the centre only for regular health visits, rather than keeping them all day at the centre. There were three types of non-treated controls: a group of nutritionally normal children, a group of malnourished children who were siblings of those in the programme and a group of malnourished children who were unrelated to the children in the programme.

Using the same outline as before, the treatments included:

Type A CSU: Cognitive stimulation, food and health care, undernourished
                children
          CSN: Cognitive stimulation, food and health care, "normal"
                children from the same neighbourhood
Type B LS: Food and health care only, undernourished children staying
                at home
Type C CO: Non-treated controls, malnourished children unrelated to
                programme children
          COS: Non-treated controls, malnourished siblings of programme
                children
          CON: Non-treated controls, "normal" children from the same
                neighbourhood

Results of this second pilot study can be summarized as follows:
  (1) The "food only" (LS) group did not fare better than controls in terms
      of psychological development. Also there seemed to be no "spill-over"
      or "diffusion" effects of the programme at home.
  (2) Other major results are related to the differences between normally
      nourished treatment children and malnourished treatment children on
      the Sentence Completion and other verbal cognitive tasks. As is to be
      expected, the normally nourished (CSN) were superior to the
      malnourished (CSU) group at the start of the programme. Also, after
      receiving the same treatment, the former maintained their superior
      position. In the five-month period of this study, however, the
      malnourished children were able to surpass the level of the normally
      nourished, poor children (CON) who received no treatment.
  (3) In non-verbal cognitive development, represented by the Knox Cubes
      data (Fig. 4), a somewhat similar relationship exists. The CSN group
      starts out higher but the CSU group catches up; not surpassing,
      however, the CON group. Considering all non-verbal tests together,
      the CSU children make gains over both CSN and CON children.

These interactions suggest that some abilities are depressed by nutritional
deficit, and may fully recover with treatment, while others may directly reflect
experiences. That is, retardations of those capabilities demanded by the non-
verbal tasks may be overcome, but the amount of information processed will
continue to reflect differences in experiential history.

The results of the two pilot studies led us to questions related to our concern
for the *relevance* of the treatment and of our measures. The stimulated and
fed undernourished children made gains over the controls. To what extent

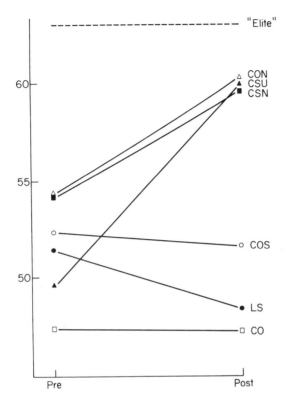

Fig. 4. Knox Cubes test score changes over the five-month period of the second pilot study. Test scores are standard scores. (CSU = cognitive stimulation, food and health care, malnourished children; CSN = cognitive stimulation, food and health care "normal" children from the same neighbourhood; LS = food and health care only, malnourished children; CO = non-treated controls, malnourished children unrelated to programme children; COS = non-treated controls, malnourished siblings of programme children; CON = non-treated controls, "normal" children from the same neighbourhood). From (4).

did this bring them close to what could be considered adequate levels of functioning for their ages? If the central purposes of the treatments are to achieve a practical, significant advantage from the treatment, then gains over non-treated controls is a significant, but unsatisfactory finding. The treated children eventually did better on the cognitive tests than the mean of their non-treated, malnourished peers from the same community. Is this adequate? What would non-malnourished, poor children do in the same circumstances?

In this second pilot study we also introduced measurements to evaluate the social–affective or social–emotional development of these children. A

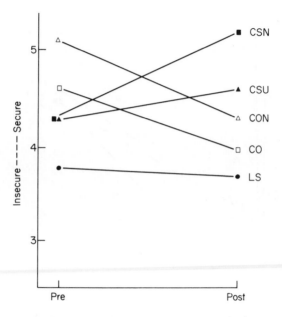

Fig. 5. Changes in rated insecurity of children over the five-month period of the second pilot study. Score units are group mean ratings on seven points rating scale. (CSU = cognitive stimulation, food and health care, malnourished children; CSN = cognitive stimulation, food and health care "normal" children from the same neighbourhood; LS = food and health care only, malnourished children; CO = non-treated controls, malnourished children unrelated to programme children; CON = non-treated controls, "normal" children from the same neighbourhood). From (4).

scale of Security–Insecurity (Fig. 5) was completed, as well as a scale for measurement of Active–Passive attitudes (Fig. 6). We were very careful in the methodology for assigning of subjects to observers, since observation of affective and social behaviour is notoriously subject to observer biases.

The Security–Insecurity scale included facial expressions, approach versus avoidance responses, and vacillation versus consistency of response tendency. The results showed the control groups moving toward the insecurity corner, while the treated groups suggested some improvement of their level of security. The food only group (LS) showed some kind of random fluctuation, although this occurred within the framework of a completely uniform relationship of treated to untreated children.

In the Active–Passive dimension (Fig. 6), the LS group moved in the same direction as the stimulated groups (CSU and CSN), while untreated controls (CO and CON) moved toward more passive attitudes in the five-month period.

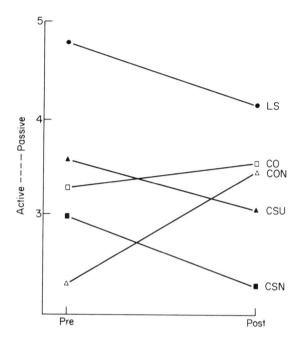

Fig. 6. Changes in rated activity of children over the five-month period of the second pilot study. Score units are group mean ratings. (CSU = cognitive stimulation, food and health care, malnourished children; CSN = cognitive stimulation, food and health care "normal" children from the same neighbourhood; LS = food and health care only, malnourished children; CO = non-treated controls, malnourished children unrelated to programme children; CON = non-treated controls, "normal" children from the same neighbourhood). From (4).

Although tentative, these data indicated to us that changes in the affective–social realm could be the most fundamental ones resulting from nutritional recuperation, even without behavioural intervention. It would appear to be a reasonable assumption that increasing the physiological *potency* of the child, and removing distracting sensory stimulation resulting from infection and disease, lays down a basis for directed responsive capacity which is more favourable to the child's receptivity for learning.

Conclusions of the two pilot studies

As a result of the two pilot projects, undertaken as a preparation for the major longitudinal project, at least two important conclusions emerged, as well as several fundamental questions. The first conclusion was that many psychological characteristics and capabilities are retarded in the first years of life in children who have chronic nutrition and other health deficits.

The second conclusion was that carefully designed experiments show that some retarded developmental characteristics are remediable through treatment beginning in the preschool years.

Third, the malnourished children were only able to catch up to their neighbourhood peers who were not malnourished, but they were still behind the "standard" of well-nourished, economically well-to-do children.

Fundamental questions raised are:

(1) What are the specific aspects of development affected by the deficits, and to what degree are they differentially affected? Especially lacking were indications of which emotional, attentional, and social behaviours are negatively affected.
(2) How relevant are these specific aspects to the future functioning of the child in school and other significant environments, in terms of the child's potential to fulfil productive and satisfying social roles?
(3) Which of the relevant behavioural capabilities and characteristics are remediable in the preschool years?
(4) With what combinations of nutritional, health, and behavioural treatments can the specific and relevant characteristics be modified positively?
(5) At what age must treatment start and for how long must it continue to provide maximum remediation of society's less favoured children?

Our longitudinal research project

Once our scientific group put together all the information derived from the two pilot studies, we were able to start to discuss alternatives for the experimental design of our longitudinal intervention programme (7). To be sure of the validity of the study, it was mandatory to adopt a model of intervention to assess direct treatment effects through nutritional supplementation, behavioural stimulation, and health care (Table 1).

At the time we started our programme, it was particularly interesting to evaluate the duration factor, which had so far been neglected. We systematically increased the duration of the multidisciplinary treatments to levels not previously reported and established evaluation results with measures directly comparable across all levels. This was done not only to test the hypothesis that longer treatments could produce greater and more enduring intellectual gains, but also to develop an appraisal of what results could be expected at different points along a continuum of action. This second

Table 1. Experimental design of the longitudinal Cali project. From (10).

Groups	N(1971)	Treatment years				N(1974)
		1971	1972	1973	1974	
T4	60	enh	enh	enh	enh	53
T3	60		enh	enh	enh	50
T2	60			enh	enh	51
T1	60				enh	50
HS	60	Upper class comparison group				52
T1 (a)	20	nh	nh	nh	enh	16
T1 (b)	20		nh	nh	enh	17
T1 (c)	20			nh	enh	16
	360					315

e = education; n = nutritional supplementation; h = health care.

objective, in addition to its intrinsic scientific interest, was projected to have another benefit; that of being useful in the practical application of early childhood programmes in the private and public sectors.

A group of 60 children from families also living in Cali, within the same range of birth-dates as the experimental group, and having a high socioeconomic status (HS), was included in the study. The idea was to have available a set of local reference standards for "normal" physical and psychological development, and not depend solely on foreign standards. Our assumption was that, in relation to available ecnomic resources, housing, food, health care, and educational opportunities, these children had the highest possibility of any group in that society for full intellectual and physical development. Though this group received no treatment in relation to the research programme, the majority were in fact attending the best private preschool nurseries during the study. They were medically and psychologically assessed at the same intervals as the treated children (Fig. 7).

Other characteristics of our work during the longitudinal intervention programme are described in *Improving Cognitive Ability in Chronically Deprived Children* (7). It is important, however, to highlight one aspect of the programme which received only passing attention in the original publication due to limitations of space, and this is the differences between the two groups in terms of SES (Table 2). The educational level (14·5 years for fathers, and 10·4 years for mothers) of the privileged group is obviously the reason for the much higher income (95%) and explains the better diet and the consequent deficient weight and height of the less privileged group of children in the experiment. It is also interesting to point out that mothers of the HS group added 1·2 years of formal education to their average during the four years of operation of the programme; a large number of them were attending the university while the programme was in progress.

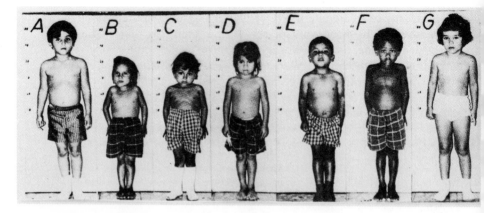

Fig. 7. Children of the longitudinal research project, 1972. (A and G = reference children; all children are four years old.) From Sinisterra, L. (1978) La ecología del desarrollo humano: ampliación del impacto de la educación médica. *Bol. Of. Sanit. Panam* **LXXXV** (4), Octubre.

Table 2. Characteristics of the experimental families in the longitudinal study. Sinisterra, L. (1978). From La ecología del desarrollo humano: ampliación del impacto de la educación médica. *Bol. Of. Sanit. Panam.* **LXXXV** (4) Octubre.

Socioeconomic characteristics	Reference group[a] ($Nq = 60$)	Experimental group[b] ($Nq = 300$)
Number of persons in house	4·9	7·5
Years education of father	14·5	3·3
Years education of mother	10·4	3·0
Total monthly income (in US $)	560	44
Persons per sleep room	1·2	4·7
Electricity or gas for cooking	100%	6%
Potable water at home	100%	4%

[a] Upper class children. [b] Lower class children.

Finally, the potential implications and the psychological consequences of the so-called assortative mating are very clear in these two groups of high and low SES. To this respect Jensen (8) states "mate selection is greatly aided by the highly visible selective process of the educational system and occupational hierarchy". Implications of assortative mating on intelligence of the progeny is also discussed by Bereiter (9). Our high SES group registered 14·5 years for fathers and 10·4 for mothers, this average increasing during the course of the programme; on the other hand, the low SES group had 3·3 years of education for fathers and 3·0 years for mothers and, for obvious reasons, this remained constant during the period studied.

Effects of treatment during the longitudinal study. During the preschool phase of the study, the integrated treatment resulted in significant gains in general cognitive ability. Figure 8 shows the progress in cognitive development among the different experimental groups and in comparison with the upper-class group. In this graph, the data for group T1 are combined with those for groups T1 (a, b, c) since they participated in only one period of integrated treatment. Several facts stand out:

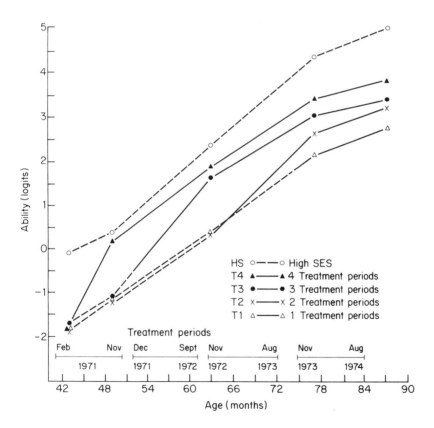

Fig. 8. Growth of general cognitive ability of study children from 43 to 87 months of age, the beginning of primary school. From (7).

(1) The effects of the treatment periods, varying in number from one to four, are cumulative: the greater the number of treatment periods, the higher the average level of cognitive ability at the end of the preschool period (87 months of age).

(2) The greatest changes in the velocity of cognitive development occur during the first treatment period.

(3) The earlier in the child's life the integrated treatment is provided, the larger are the effects during the first treatment period. Physical growth shows the same tendency but less clearly.

(4) After the first treatment period, the gap between the mean performance scores of the children of the comparison group (HS: high socioeconomic status, untreated) and the experimental groups (low socioeconomic and nutritional status, treated) has been widening.

Results of the initial two years of follow-up (10). We were able to follow-up the children who participated in our longitudinal project for the following two years while all of them were going to the public schools in Cali. Figure 9 portrays cognitive development during the first two years of school, following the cessation of experimental intervention at the end of the preschool period. The experimental groups (T1 to T4) maintain their position relative to each other but there is a levelling off in intellectual performance, while the HS group exhibited continued growth. The gap between the children of high and low socioeconomic status became still wider.

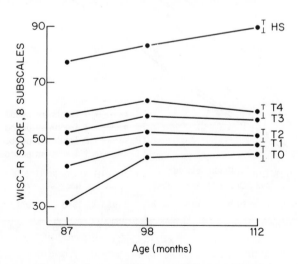

Fig. 9. Progress of cognitive development of experimental and comparison groups in the period following preschool intervention. From (10).

Group T0 (low socioeconomic status, untreated) first tested at the end of the preschool period, has the lowest performance level. The score at 87 months may be depressed, in part, because they had no previous experience in taking tests. By 112 months of age this initial disadvantage has probably been overcome. The fact that children in the T0 group were, at least initially, the healthiest and physically most normal children, and yet show scores lower than the least treated group, leads us to conclude that strong obstacles to normal cognitive growth in the urban poverty environment exist even when nutritional conditions are not grossly inadequate.

The physical work capacity of our study children. Physical work capacity is best measured by the maximum oxygen consumption (V_{O_2} max) and has been markedly depressed by undernutrition. Barac-Nieto *et al.* (11) have shown that the V_{O_2} max is progressively lower in subjects with increasing severity of undernutrition.

Spurr and co-workers (12) have reported their findings in Colombian sugar cane cutters in whom they found a clear relationship between productivity as cane cutters and their indices of present (V_{O_2} max) or previous (height) nutritional status. They consider that undernutrition at an early age will limit the development of full genetic potential of body size (height and weight), limiting working capacity and productivity.

On that basis, this group of physiologists accepted our invitation to measure V_{O_2} max of our experimental children, comparing them with the results of the children of the upper class comparison group (Table 3). Their results are very clear and their comments very pertinent (13):

(a) Malnutrition in early life depresses growth and results in smaller adults. (b) Small adults produce less, since productivity in both light and heavy industrial work is related to body size. (c) Heavy industrial work is also related to maximum working capacity as measured by the V_{O_2} max. (c) Undernutrition early in life depressed the body size and V_{O_2} max of six-year-old children when compared to advantaged children of the same age who had not been exposed to malnutrition. (d) Three years of dietary supplementation between three and six years of age, while it improved growth, did not result in increased V_{O_2} max.

It is very interesting to consider the implications suggested by the study of the vitality of preschool children as measured by the V_{O_2} max. This limitation on available energy could be the reason for the limited physical activity and mental apathy of infants and young children from poor sectors of tropical towns. As a consequence, children will see their curiosity limited by their limited available energy, and as such their exploring and getting acquainted with the world will be also limited. All these factors will contribute to the slow mental development of poor, undernourished children.

Table 3. Means and standard deviations of anthropometry and maximum physiological responses of disadvantaged Colombian, and advantaged Colombian and American six-year-old children. From (13).

Parameter	Disadvantaged[a]			Probability[b]	Advantaged[c,d]		Probability[b]
	Group 1[e]	Group 2	Group 3	Groups 1–3	Group 4	Group 5	Groups 1–5
Body weight (kg)	17·5±1·5	16·9±1·2	15·0±1·3	<0·002	23·8±4·2	21·6±3·1	<0·0001
Height (cm)	105·6±3·0	105·7±3·2	101·8±4·3	<0·05	120·5±5·3	120·0±6·2	<0·0001
Weight/height (kg/m)	16·5±1·2	16·0±0·9	14·7±0·8	<0·002	19·7±2·9	18·0±1·7	<0·0001
Max heart rate, (beats/min)	197±11	195±9	196±10	NS	197±5	192±6	NS
V_{O_2} max (STPD), (ml/min)	603±71	584±108	500±97	<0·05	901±112	912±207	<0·0001
V_{O_2} max (STPD), (ml/kg/min)	34·6±3·7	34·5±5·6	33·2±5·0	NS	38·1±2·4	41·7±4·3	<0·01
O_2 pulse (ml/beat)	3·1±0·4	3·0±0·6	2·6±0·5	NS	4·6±0·7	4·8±1·1	<0·0001
V_E max (BTPS) (l/min)	29·7±4·9	27·5±4·7	27·1±6·6	NS	44·1±6·0	39·7±7·1	<0·0001

[a] Undernourished at age 3. [b] One way analysis of variance. [c] Never exposed to undernutrition. [d] No stastically significant difference between groups 4 and 5. [e] Group 1 — Dietary repletion at school (n=10); Group 2 — Dietary repletion at home (n=10); Group 3 — No dietary repletion (n=10); Group 4 — Colombians (n=6); Group 5 — Americans (n=6). NS = Not statistically significant.

Reanalysis of the Cali project. Bejar has carefully performed a complete reanalysis of our data. As a result he expresses (14) his purpose as being; "to assess the contribution of the nutritional intervention component relative to the contribution of the educational component of the treatment." His conclusion is very clear:

> There is, however, an important lesson to be learned from the Cali study, namely, a formula to counter the effect of a poor environment on cognitive development. The key element in that formula seems to be the educational treatment, not the nutritional supplementation . . . The Cali study provides evidence that regardless of the heritability of intelligence, environmental intervention in the form of an educational treatment has a significant impact on it.

Final Observations and Remarks

The initial purely medical and nutritional research of the scientific group of HERF made it clear that the children treated and recovered also suffered a psychological and emotional impact which limited their educational development.

For more than four years, the group applied a most elaborate and complete educational technology to groups of chronically deprived children of increasing ages at entrance to the programme: group T4 received 4170 hours of treatment; group T3 received 3130 hours; group T2, 2070 hours; and group T1, 990 hours. All the groups responded clearly to the stimulation received and in proportion to the number of hours exposed to the programme. It is also clear though that the earlier treatment begins, the better. Children entering earlier (at three years) showed a better response and longer lasting effects.

As a result of the longitudinal follow-up, the children, shortly after finishing the intervention (educational and nutritional), showed diminishing or almost disappearing gains with the passing of years, using the school performance as a criterion. It seems clear that social and educational backwardness cannot be cured by the educational and nutritional interventions of the type we used. It is true that amelioration is clearly seen, but it is also transitory . . . and its cost is so high that promoting its extension is not justifiable.

The Consequences of Scientific Research in Colombia

Last but not least, it is timely to mention the political impact which it is possible to produce through the scientific initiatives we are able to implement.

Colombia appears to be particularly sensitive to the problem of the sufferings of the less favoured children as a result of undernutrition and general social deprivation. As a consequence of the world-wide interest in the problem of human undernutrition affecting growing children, the Colombian Congress in 1969 approved Law 27 which created a special tax, equivalent to 2% of the value of the monthly payroll of private and public institutions, to be paid to the new Colombian Institute of Family Welfare (ICBF), created with the mandate to care specifically for poor pregnant women, their newborn and infants, up to the age of seven years.

In the last 15 years, ICBF has implemented the production of vegetable protein mixtures and their own brand, Bienestarina, is being widely produced and distributed everywhere in the country. It has also promoted and administered health and education centres called Centres for Integral Care of the Preschool Child (CAIP) which are giving care to more than 2 000 000 Colombian preschool children (approximately 50% of the needy children).

Present Research Plans

We are at present evaluating community responses and personal reactions from the poor sectors in Cali where its programmes are located. The interest of these human groups in the general process of child growth and development and the possibilities to improve and optimize this interest with very active adult participation are being studied. Before testing any formal scientific scheme of exploration, we have decided first to evaluate the possibilities our initiatives could have in provoking a serious personal commitment on the part of pregnant women, mothers, and families, in the implementation of a new approach to child growth and stimulation.

The experience we have so far accumulated has convinced us of the unquestionable importance of the emotional participation of the pregnant woman and later on, of the lactating mother, in the whole process of pregnancy, delivery, and nursing of the baby. To "carry" the fetus and later on to dress, undress, clean, and feed the baby is not enough. Nurturing the baby, expressing love and tenderness, is mandatory for the adequate, and even more so, for the optimal development of the child. The rest of the technical and scientific participation of the environment in fostering the child's development is evidently useful, but is insufficient.

It is worth mentioning that our current conviction of the need first to optimize the relationship between the woman and her pregnancy, and later on between the mother and her baby, before trying out any marginal intervention, derives from our certainty that all other intervention is just that: marginal in importance in the overall process of the development of the child.

A warm and solid mother–child relationship is the very backbone of the whole process and the reinvigoration of it should be the *raison d'être* of all other external intervention.

We should mention that we have found that the weak bond between the mother and the product of her conception derives mostly from ignorance: the mother's plain and absolute ignorance of every aspect of reproduction. The men tend to ignore the other half of the process and the final result of conception, particularly among underprivileged groups, is what we call a poor orphan, deprived in the emotional and psychological realm. The human species in its secular process of evolution towards becoming better and brighter has forgotten its instincts and, acting blind-folded in this important sphere of reproduction, has been misled by others whose level of ignorance is as bad or worse (15).

To try to ameliorate the situation the HERF staff have decided to gather together groups of women in the early stages of their pregnancies. Meetings are held twice a week informally to discuss everyone's version of pregnancy, reproduction, mothering, education, affection, and final child development. The staff contribute with films, pictures, and instruction on child development, and the pregnant women, in a very simple way, contribute their own experience and limited knowledge on the matter. We have probably learned more than they.

Our present, very tentative, scheme of work includes nutritional supplementation (Colombiharina) enriched with small amounts of vegetable oils — maize, sunflower and soyabean — to provide essential fatty acids, and a very strong promotion of early child stimulation, all beginning in early pregnancy and involving both father and mother. We insist on mothers gaining at least 10 kilograms of weight and suggest they gain a good part of this weight during the first half of their pregnancy (16).

We expect to accumulate enough evidence so as to be able to design experiments with intervention within the next eight months to a year. The very positive and enthusiastic participation of mothers, fathers, and the family at large, is prompting us to give more and more responsibility to them in the teaching, supervision, and actual management of some aspects of the maternal and child health and nutrition programme. Their knowledge of local foods and cooking techniques and of other important aspects is useful, but is incomplete and requires our monitoring and evaluation.

Competition between groups in relation to results such as gain of weight of mother and child, speed to learn, etc., is being promoted by the group itself. In general, the community appears to enjoy learning and living the everyday episodes of mother and child growth and development.

Finally, a programme of maternal and child health, nutrition, and development should be considered part of the Community Development programme, and should involve the community, the government, the university, and all the liberal professions who care and can participate in the supervision and quality control of a programme that enhances potential of the human being by offering him the possibilities instead of the limitations of life.

References

1. Population Reference Bureau, Inc. (1983). Crecimiento de las ciudades latinoamericanas. *INTERCOM* **4**, 3:5.
2. Sinisterra, L. (1969). A vegetable protein mixture for the prevention and treatment of preschool malnutrition: Colombiharina. Paper presented at the VIII International Nutrition Congress, Prague, 1969.
3. Ghitis, J., Velez, H., Linares, F., Sinisterra, L. and Vitale, J. (1963). The erithroid atrophy in kwashiorkor and Marasmus: Cali-Harvard Nutrition Project, L. Sinisterra, Director. *Am. J. Clin. Nutr.* **12**, 445–451.
4. McKay, H. E., McKay, A. and Sinisterra, L. (1973). Behavioral intervention studies with malnourished children: a review of experiences. *In* "Nutrition, Development, and Social Behavior" (D. J. Kallen, ed.) pp. 121–145. US Department of Health Education and Welfare, Publication No. (NIH) 73–242.
5. Riecken, H. and Boruch R. (eds.) (1974). "Social Experimentation. A Method for Planning and Evaluating Social Intervention," pp. 88, 104, 125, 309, and 330. Academic Press, New York.
6. Jelliffe, D. B. (1966). "The Assessment of the Nutritional Status of the Community," pp. 10–96. World Health Organization, Geneva.
7. McKay, H., Sinisterra, L., McKay, A., Gómez, H. and Lloreda, P. (1978). Improving cognitive ability in chronically deprived children. *Science* **200**, 270–278.
8. Jensen, A. R. "How Much Can We Boost IQ and Scholastic Achievement?" Reprint Series No. 2, Environment, Heredity and Intelligence. pp. 1–117. *Educational Review*, Boston.
9. Bereiter, C. (1969). "The Future of Individual Differences." Reprint Series No. 2, Environment, Heredity and Intelligence, pp. 162–170. *Harvard Educational Review*, Boston.
10. Sinisterra, L., McKay, H., McKay, A., Gómez, H. and Korgi, J. (1979). Response of malnourished school children to multidisciplinary intervention. *In* "Proceedings of the International Nutrition Conference: Behavioral Effects of Energy and Protein Deficits" (J. Brožek, ed.) pp. 229–238. US Department of Health Education and Welfare, NIH Publication No. 79–1906.
11. Barac-Nieto, M., Spurr, G. B., Maksud, M. G. and Lotero, H. (1978). Aerobic capacity in chronically undernourished adult males. *J. App. Physiol.* **44** (2), 209–215.
12. Spurr, G. B., Barac-Nieto, M., Maksud, M. G. and Lotero, H. (1977). Productivity and maximal oxygen consumption in sugarcane cutters. *Am. J. Clin. Nutr.* **30**, 316–321.
13. Spurr, G. B., Barac-Nieto, M. and Maksud, M. G. (1978). Childhood undernutrition: implications for adult work capacity and productivity. *In* "Environmental Stress: Individual Human Adaptations", Section III, (L. J. Folinsbee, *et al.* eds) pp. 165–181. Academic Press, New York.
14. Bejar, I. (1981). Does nutrition cause intelligence? A reanalysis of the Cali experiment. *Intelligence* **5**, 49–68.

15. Dobbing, J. (1984). Breast is best, isn't it? *In* "Health Hazards of Milk" (D. L. J. Freed, ed.) pp. 60–74. Bailliere Tindall, London.
16. Hytten, F. E. and Thomson, M. (1975). Ajustes Fisiológicos Maternos. *In* "Nutrición de la Futura Madre y Evolución del Embarazo". Committee on Maternal Nutrition, Food and Nutrition Board, National Research Board, National Academy of Sciences. Editorial Limusa, México, pp. 53–86.

Acknowledgements

The research group would like to acknowledge in particular the helpful advice of Drs Fernando Monckeberg, John W. McDavid and David P. Weikart throughout the longitudinal study.

Commentary

I. Hurwitz: This report begins with an all too familiar and grim account of the urbanization of developing countries in Latin America. The consequences of overcrowding, inadequate housing, poor sanitation, insufficient medical and health care and poor nutrition continue to create a picture in which the prospects for finding meaningful and effective long-term intervention and remediation become increasingly diminished. Those with the highest degree of vulnerability to these poor conditions, specifically women and children, seem faced with the almost inevitable outcomes of intellectual, emotional and social disabilities in the face of grinding poverty. Even with nutritionally based interventions, (supplementation, etc.) the author reports a Sisyphis-like process in which temporary improvement is consistently followed by relapse in individual cases, and an increase in the numbers of new cases. It becomes clear that relying only on nutritional supplementation, "repeatedly proved to be excellent for physical recuperation", is "useless in the face of the mental impact of malnutrition and chronic deprivation".

The chapter then presents us with an account of a series of studies which increasingly focusses on efforts to identify what cognitive, social and emotional factors were more susceptible to the effects of undernutrition and malnutrition, and which types of interventions were more efficacious in correcting these problems, particularly with respect to the timing and duration of the poor nutrition.

With respect to the initial pilot study, results centre on the observations, first, that the Knox Cube and Sentence Memory Test showed no positive differential in the performance of treated and control groups in favour of the former, and second, the lack of advantage of cognitive stimulation over physical stimulation, i.e. emphasizing verbal over motor activity as remedial programmes failed to bring about different outcome effects. The two former measures are identified as assessing short-term memory, although it would be this writer's contention that an even more basic issue is involved, namely that of attentional processes. Barrett's studies (1) indicate that "distractibility and inattentiveness (are) found in all school age subjects malnourished in infancy", a finding corroborated by Mora *et al.* (2), and Chavez and Martinez (3), by Lester (4) in studies of infants and toddlers, and by Keys *et al.* (5) in starving adults. This distinction between attentional deficits on the one hand, and memory processes on the other, may be important from the standpoint of remediation, since both pharmacological and educational rehabilitative programmes may be more accurately and effectively aimed at basic attentional deficits rather than at correcting "memory impairment", a problem area which may be a good deal more complex than "attention" in the sequence of activities in the learning process.

With respect to the lack of apparent advantage of cognitive, i.e. verbal stimulation over physical stimulation, the latter defined as "a high peak of daily motor activity", this result may be understood in terms of developmental theory which postulates that at early ages, experiences are more likely to be fused into syncretic unities so that *all* stimulation, whether motor or cognitive, may provide a non-specific activating or energizing role in the developing young child, affecting a common substrate out of which such specific functions as verbal skills and other particular competencies may eventually differentiate. Furthermore, one cannot exclude the perhaps obvious possibility that heightened motor activity has the effect of actually exposing the child to a broader range of exteroceptive stimulation as well as increasing the flow of internal kinaesthetic and proprioceptive impulses, which may collectively serve to organize and enhance body awareness and positive body image.

The second "pilot study" described in this paper concluded that, in general, non-verbal skills seem recoverable while verbal competence, essential for processing information, "will continue to reflect the differences [between rehabilitated, undernourished populations living in poverty and well-nourished children of comfortable backgrounds] in experiential history".

Sinisterra adds that the question of relevance of behaviours and functions assumes major importance where relevance attaches to the meaning of broad developmental issues in "social–affective" and "social–emotional" areas of growth and change. This concern led these researchers to the "one to four year" longitudinal study, a well-controlled assessment of the effects of nutritional, medical, and cognitive interventions.* The outcomes of the longitudinal study are not surprising with regard to the effects of intervention programmes of longer duration on cognitive ability, though the well-nourished and economically better off group shows a continuously accelerated growth curve. The entire thrust of the outcome is best stated by Sinisterra's own quote of Bejar's comment:

> The key element seems to be the educational treatment, not the nutritional supplementation, regardless of the heritability of intelligence, environmental intervention in the form of an educational treatment has a significant impact on it.

The conclusions of this study, reached after literally thousands of hours of intervention had been devoted to the care of the children involved, nevertheless led the investigators to another even more significant realization, namely that effective intervention had to begin with the attitude, feelings expectations and skills of the expectant mother. One could see in Sinisterra's comments the long shadow of early experiments evaluating the quality of early mother-child attachment processes initiated more than three decades ago in the work of Bowlby (9) and the Robertsons (10), and leading to more recent studies by Ainsworth (11), Caldwell (12), Papousek (13), Osofsky (14), and Barrett (15). The delicate, vital, and yet easily neglected area of early parenting, by both mother and father, can be forgotten in our headlong search for technological sophistication, and in our awe of the computer, the machine, and the quantifiable, measurable index of physical or biological variables. The characters of the mother-to-child, father-to-child, child-to-mother and child-to-father interactions, in spite of all the vagueness, uncertainty, ambiguity, and elusiveness that exist around these variables, still represent the essential foundation upon which the effects of virtually all influences on the child, positive as well as negative, from meaningful sensory stimulation and physical activity, to the grim impact of malnutrition and undernutrition, can be best understood. It is very likely that it is this process which holds the key to the success or failure of both nutritional and educational programmes.

I find it is necessary to comment on a statement made in this report, "It is not the function of scientists to change the economic and political structure of a society, but it is our responsibility to understand its inequalities and limitations because it is within this context that we must exercise our

---

* It is interesting to note the reference made by Sinisterra to the advanced level of education of both mothers and fathers in the well-nourished, high socioeconomic status control families, and the low and even declining levels in the poorer populations. He invokes the distasteful and discredited notions of Jensen, with their implications for a kind of biological fixity to "intelligence" as a heritable factor, the low level of which, in the undernourished group, is supposedly perpetuated by "assortive mating", that is that uneducated, and therefore, by inference, unintelligent people, will produce unintelligent offspring. (See ref. 8 for a discussion of this issue.)

knowledge." If the "inequalities and limitations" refer to the differential skills and knowledge available to scientists on the one hand, but unknown to society in general on the other, I would agree. However, if this phrase refers to the inequalities and limitations of society which create poverty and suffering, then I would submit that the scientist must devote a sizeable proportion of his/her energies to supporting political and economic change. Indeed, it is precisely this that scientists are in an advantageous position to foster and bring about. The treatment of approximately 300 children in four years in the Cali studies is certainly a laudable effort in principle and in its execution, but even more important is what Sinisterra alludes to as an obligation of science in his closing paragraph, namely that:

> A programme of maternal and child health nutrition, and development should . . . involve the community, the government, the university and all the liberal professions who care and can participate in a programme that enhances potential of the human being by offering him the possibilities instead of the limitations of life.

To this I would add that vigorous demands upon government, when exerted by the scientific community, should result not in the "offering of possibilities," but in the assuring of realities!

1. Barrett, D. E. (1984). Malnutrition and Child Behavior. *In* "Malnutrition and Behavior: A Critical Assessment of Key Issues" (J. Brožek and B. Schürch, eds) Nestlé Foundation, Lausanne, Switzerland.
2. Mora, J. O., Clement, J., Christianten, N., Ortiz, N., Vuori, L. and Wagner, M. (1979). Nutritional supplementation, early stimulation and child development. *In* "Behavior Effects of Protein and Energy Deficits" (J. Brožek, ed.) DHEW Publ. No. 79–106, Washington, DC.
3. Chavez, A. and Martinez C. (1979). Consequences of insufficient nutrition on child character and behavior. *In* "Malnutrition, Environment and Behavior". Cornell University Press, Ithaca, NY.
4. Lester, B. M. (1975). Cardiac habituation of the orienting response of infants of varying nutritional states. *Devl Psychol.* **11**, 432–442.
5. Keys, S. A., Brožek, J., Henschel, A., Mickelson, O. and Taylor, H. (1950). "The Biology of Human Starvation," Vol. 11. University of Minnesota Press, Minneapolis, MN.
6. Fraňková, S. and Barnes, R. H. (1973). Effect of protein calorie malnutrition on the development of social behavior in rats. *Devl Psychobiol.* **6**, 33–43.
7. Jensen, A. (1969). How much can we boost IQ and scholastic achievement? *Harvard Educational Review* **39**, 1–123, Cambridge, MA.
8. Gould, S. J. (1983). "The Mismeasure of Man." W. W. Norton, New York.
9. Bowlby, J. (1960). Separation anxiety. *Int. J. Psychoanal.* **41**, 69–113.
10. Robertson J. (1958). "Young Children in Hospital." Tavistock Publications, Inc. London.
11. Ainsworth, M. D. S. and Bell, S. M. (1969). Some contemporary patterns of mother–infant interactions in the feeding situation. *In* "Stimulation in Early Infants" (J. A. Ambrose, ed.). Academic Press, London.

12. Caldwell, B. M. (1962). Assessment of infant personality. *Merrill-Palmer Q. Behav. Dev.* **2**, 71–81.
13. Papousek, H. (1967). Experimental studies of appetitional behavior in human newborns. *In* "Early Behavior: Comparative and Developmental Approaches" (H. W. Stevenson, E. H. Hess and H. L. Rheingold, eds). John Wiley & Sons, New York.
14. Osofsky, J. D. (1976). Neonatal characteristics and maternal infant interaction in two observational situations. *Child Dev.* **47**, 1138–1147.
15. Barrett, D. E., *op cit.*

Sally Grantham-McGregor: Sinisterra reports a very important series of studies, which have contributed immensely to our knowledge of child development.

As far as addressing the question of whether malnutrition affects mental development and later achievement, it must be remembered that these studies only addressed the question of whether the mental development of children who were already undernourished is rehabilitated with improved nutrition. This may not be the same as giving nutritional supplementation from birth and preventing the occurrence of malnutrition.

It would be most helpful to see the figures for the nutritional status of the groups of children before and after intervention for each study. In particular, it is critical to know the exact degree of improvement in nutritional status which was not associated with concurrent improvement in mental development.

The somewhat older age of the children in these studies may be an important factor in the failure to find a benefit to mental development from nutritional supplementation alone.

The two pilot studies which are referred to are fascinating; however it would be nice to see more details of the findings. I have been unable to locate them in the published literature except in a preliminary report (1). The duration of the pilot studies was short and I wonder what is the mechanism postulated for improved nutrition leading to improved mental development in four or five months.

For improvement in activity level in the group which only received improved nutrition and health care in the second pilot study is an important finding and poses the question of whether or not increased activity is related to improved cognitive functioning. In this particular case it was not, but perhaps the time period was too short for an association to manifest itself. It would be helpful to know how the activity rating was constructed.

The second pilot study is also of special interest because there was a normal group participating in intervention. Although they maintain their initial advantage at the post-intervention test in some areas, the intervened malnourished children actually catch up to the intervened "normals" in other areas.

This suggests a greater response to intervention in malnourished children than in better nourished children; however it may be a plateau or ceiling effect. It would be most valuable to have a closer look at the data.

Sinisterra lists some important questions. We may add: What particular disadvantages affect which aspects of development?

1. McKay, H. E., McKay, A. and Sinisterra, L. (1973). Behavioural intervention studies with malnourished children: a review of experiences. *In* "Nutrition, Development and Social Behavior" (D. J. Kallen, ed.) pp. 121–146. US Department of Health Education and Welfare, Publication No. (NIH) 73–242.

K. S. Bedi: Sinisterra describes some "intervention" studies (also reviewed in the chapter by Grantham-McGregor) where he has examined malnourished children in Cali (Colombia). In these studies he essentially had three groups. The first consisted of malnourished children who were given nutritional supplement and health care, as well as behavioural stimulation. The second group were only given nutritional supplement and health care, whilst the third group were not given any treatment at all. For obvious ethical reasons there were no children who received the behavioural stimulation but not the nutritional supplementation.

In the first pilot study the "no treatment" children were the siblings of the treated children. Is it considered ethical to give some children nutritional supplement while deliberately denying their malnourished brothers and sisters the same supplement? In any case, do siblings make "good" controls under such circumstances? Giving one child in a family nutritional supplementation may also result in more food being available for the other members of the family, simply because the family has one fewer "mouth to feed".

Sinisterra's studies also attempted to differentiate between types (e.g. cognitive or physical) as well as degrees (e.g. high or low) of stimulation. Is it really possible to give cognitive stimulation without also giving some physical stimulation? In addition, whether the degree of stimulation was high or low was really only a subjective classification on the part of the researchers. Because of the multifactorial design of Sinisterra's studies, in addition to the lack of all the necessary controls, it can be argued that the conclusions reached are rather tentative.

Turning now more specifically to the longitudinal study, Sinisterra examined the effects of varying the period and duration of the nutritional supplementation, health care and stimulation ("integrated treatment") on general cognitive ability. Figure 8 shows graphs of the cognitive ability scores versus the age of five groups of children. One of these groups consisted of children from high income families. The remaining groups contained malnourished children who had been given 1, 2, 3 or 4 periods of the integrated treatment. The malnourished children seemed to improve their cognitive ability scores with increasing age. Those given the longer treatment periods appear to do slightly better than those who received shorter periods of treatments, although they never reached the same levels as the children from the high income families. Whether this apparent "catch-up" in cognitive ability was real or not remains uncertain as the statistical analyses of the interactions are not presented.

Author's reply: We were always very careful about ethics. Children receiving food always received it in our centre, several blocks away from their homes. When we sent food to their homes, we always sent food for *all* the members of the family: the 60 children receiving food only in fact entailed providing food for 238 people in the final year. This made our programme particularly expensive, but that is how we had decided to do it.

Those children receiving food at home, both for themselves and the rest of the family, were the children studied as controls for physical and mental development. They gained weight and height as much as the children participating in the centre's comprehensive programme (nutrition, medical care and education), but their mental progress was as retarded as that of the total controls who entered the comprehensive programme only at the age of six.

The use of siblings in pilot studies 1 and 2 was during the initial days (1969–70) when we were testing how children in these particular communities grew and made mental progress when they received food and educational stimulus, compared with their brothers and sisters at home. The food and stimulus were always given in our centre. In these pilot studies, which lasted 4–5 months, we were basically making the administrative and cost evaluations indispensible for the writing of our initial grant proposal.

J. L. Smart: Given the enormous cost of the kinds of intervention employed in Sinisterra's study, it might have been useful to have asked a sixth "Fundamental question" in the definitive study:

(6) What type of intervention at which age results in the greatest benefit per unit cost?

From this point of view it would have been better to concentrate treatment groups on the youngest rather than the oldest ages (Table 1). In particular, it would have been interesting to follow the progress of a group treatment in the earliest year (1971) only.

The progress of cognitive development, as reflected in WISC scores, is interesting (Fig. 9). I assume that the scores are standardized for age and that the "expected" developmental profile for a group of children is a straight, horizontal line. All six groups in the Cali study improve between 87 and 98 months of age, though this might merely reflect increasing familiarity with the test. Only the high socioeconomic group (HS) continued to improve between 98 and 112 months, but the other groups, with the possible exception of the longest intervention group (T4), maintained their scores at their 98-month level. Hence, it may be unduly pessimistic to conclude that ". . . amelioration is clearly seen but it is also transitory. . .".

I was pleased to see that in an offshoot of the main investigation a physiological measure of functional capacity was measured, namely V_{O_2} max. I am no expert in this field and hence I have little idea whether it is more meaningful to express V_{O_2} max per whole individual or per kilogram body weight. Perhaps the experts are also unsure, since I notice that this measure is expressed both ways in Table 3. The conclusion that "Three years of dietary supplementation between three and six years of age, which improved growth, did not result in increased V_{O_2} max," must be based on V_O max per kg body weight for which there was no significant difference between supplemented and non-supplemented children. However, V_{O_2} max per child was higher in the supplemented children (Table 3). Again I feel that the conclusion errs on the side of pessimism.

D. E. Barrett: Sinisterra's paper raises several questions. My major question is, why, given the great concern with "a greater variety of behavioural measurement" to measure "affective, attentional, social and other non-cognitive characteristics", the investigators made only two measurements of child emotional characteristics or social behaviour, and these using procedures of questionable reliability and validity.

In introducing the pilot studies, Sinisterra states as his primary measurement objective, "identifying the specific aspects of psychological development retarded by nutritional, health and other environmental deficits". And in introducing the longitudinal research project, he said that a major question was "What are the specific aspects of development affected by the deficits . . . Especially lacking were indications of which emotional, attentional and social behaviours are negatively affected."

Given the frequent references to the need to measure social and emotional characteristics, it is surprising that in the longitudinal study there were no data reported on child social or emotional characteristics and that in the pilot studies (specifically, the second pilot study), the only measures used, at least, the only measures for which data were reported, were two rating scales (Security–Insecurity and Active–Passive), for which data on methodology are not reported and there is no basis for inferring reliability or validity of the measures.

Why was this? Was it because of the assumption that "The social–affective or social–emotional development of young children is particularly hard to measure." I don't agree with this statement, and it is not a good reason for not developing behavioural outcome variables. That is, if there are strong theoretical grounds for measuring certain aspects of the child's behaviour, and Sinisterra makes an argument for studying the effects of malnutrition on attentional and emotional characteristics, then we should try to develop and refine measures of those characteristics.

Second, I question the statement "The very complex interrelationships among health, nutrition, and family factors in the psychological development of young children can only be studied adopting an intervention model as the primary research mechanism." In fact, I believe that the only way to begin to examine the "complex interrelationships" among these factors is through naturalistic, cross-sectional research. where free-living populations are studied without intervention. The method of experimental (i.e. intervention) designs is to negate the natural dependencies between variables. By experimental control of environmental variables (i.e. selecting subjects of similar demographic characteristics and assigning them randomly to treatments) and statistical control of such variables (e.g. covarying social–demographic variables in the analysis of variance), the independent variables of interest can be isolated. Non-experimental designs, by revealing the naturally occurring relationships between health, family and nutritional influences, provide the empirical base for the experimental research (1,2).

I have two other comments, both concerning the contributions of this work.

First, I think that is the only major intervention study which *both* (a) examines combined effects between nutritional and educational intervention variables as they affect children's development, and (b) studies the effects of such factors for preschool age children. Thus, the study addresses theoretical and social questions not previously addressed, and it makes a contribution to the literature on preschool intervention for disadvantaged children (3,4).

Second, I believe Sinisterra is correct in his statement that understanding the parent–child relationship is critical if we are studying the development of the child. In nutritional intervention research we should attempt to study the effects of our intervention(s) on the mother–child relationship. In my chapter in this volume I suggest a developmental framework for developing measures of maternal responsiveness to the child for research on malnutrition and behaviour.

1. Barrett, D. E. (1984). Methodological requirements for conceptually valid research studies on the behavioral effects of malnutrition. *In* "Nutrition and Behavior" (J. R. Galler, ed.) pp. 9–36. Plenum Press, New York.
2. Barrett, D. E. (1984). Methodological issues in nutritional intervention research. *In* "Malnutrition and Behavior: A Critical Assessment of Key Issues" (J. Brožek and B. Schürch, eds) pp. 585–596. Nestlé Foundation, Lausanne, Switzerland.

3. Lazar, I. and Darlington, R. (1982). Lasting effects of early education: A report from the Consortium of Longitudinal Studies. *Monogr. Soc. Res. Child Devel.* **47** (2–3 Serial No. 195).
4. Zigler, E. and Berman, W. (1983). Discerning the future of early childhood education. *Am. Psychol.* **38**, 894–906.

D. A. Levitsky and Barbara J. Strupp: Despite such an impressive approach to the problem, the results from the two pilot studies and the preliminary results of the longitudinal study are disappointing. This disappointment stems from the Cali group's observations that the benefit of providing supplemental nutrition and environmental therapy to poor and malnourished children was so small and temporary. In order to understand why the outcome of their treatment was so small, we must examine not merely the methodologies employed by these researchers, but also the fundamental assumptions an concepts that underlie their research.

The basic premise underlying the Cali group's research is that "Environmental Deprivation is a major factor in the aetiology of the long-term effects of early malnutrition". Historically, it is important to recall that this Environmental Deprivation model was an optimistic alternative explanation to the more pessimistic "brain damage" model of malnutrition and cognitive development that was so prominent in the 1960s. Its optimism grew from the possibility that if Environmental Deprivation was the cause of the poor cognitive deficits seen in malnourished children, rather than permanent brain damage, then it should be possible to facilitate the intellectual recovery of these children to the level of non-malnourished children by providing them with Environmental Stimulation (Enrichment).

Unfortunately, such optimistic deductions from this hypothesis blinded the Cali group, as well as most of the researchers in the area, including ourselves, to some fundamental problems with Environmental Deprivation Hypothesis. The most basic problem with the conception is the fact that the Deprivation Hypothesis cannot be disproved because it cannot be scientifically tested. In order to disprove the Environmental Deprivation Hypothesis, it is necessary to examine the effects of malnutrition in two groups of humans (or animals) that have had identical experience. But because exposure to malnutrition produces a unique experience, it is impossible to ever create or devise a non-malnourished control group having exactly the same experience as the malnourished group.

This particular criticism of the Environmental Deprivation Hypothesis neither invalidates the work by the Cali group nor explains their weak effects. It merely points out a weakness in the theoretical framework upon which their therapy is built. However, the examination of other implications of the Environmental Deprivation Hypothesis applies more directly. One subtle implication of the Environmental Deprivation Hypothesis is that malnourished children (or animals) acquire very little cognitive information about the world around them. They are conceived as remaining in a suspended state of intellectual growth. Consequently, the recovery process is perceived as a method of restoring the deprived items to the organism: nutrients and cognitive information.

There is reason to believe, however, that learning and cognitive growth does continue during the period of malnutrition. There presently exists almost no evidence clearly demonstrating that even the most severe malnutrition interferes with the basic ability of either an animal or a child to learn. This statement does not mean that malnourished animals or children learn the same kinds of information from their environment as their well-nourished counterparts, merely that there is little evidence to believe that learning and cognitive growth are not continuing in malnourished organisms.

The degree to which children learn about their environment during the time they are malnourished, affects how they will respond to programmes of cognitive stimulation during nutritional rehabilitation. If malnourished children learn information that is contrary to what is being taught in programmes of cognitive stimulation, then before these children could maximally benefit from the programme, they must first *unlearn* contradictory information.

What could a malnourished child learn that would be contrary to optimal cognitive development? One possibility is the concept of control. Whereas well-nourished, healthy children may learn that they can exert considerable control over their environment through actively playing, manipulating and interacting with objects and other organisms in their environment, poorly nourished children may learn just the opposite. Malnourished children find themselves in a situation in which they cannot relieve their suffering. Such conditions are ideal for teaching children the concept of "learned helplessness" (1). Learning helplessness may be further facilitated by the children learning that an effective strategy for surviving in a situation with limited caloric intake is to minimize their interaction with the environment. Such interactions require energy and will increase the drain on their limited energy resources.

This interpretation of the effects of malnutrition on children is reinforced by the observation of the Cali group that children suffering mild degrees of malnutrition felt more insecure than their well-nourished controls (Fig. 5), and were considerably more passive (Fig. 6). Both characteristics would impede the acquisition of the information provided in the cognitive enrichment programmes. More importantly, if the children return to the same conditions that initially caused the malnutrition after terminating the enrichment programme, it would be reasonable to expect the children to return to those same responses that enabled them to survive in their environment (helplessness) and the effects of the enrichment programme would extinguish, as indicated by Fig. 9.

Though disappointing, the failure of the Cali group to demonstrate long-term effects of cognitive interventions in children is very similar to the observation of others. Like the Cali group, other investigations have found the effects of early cognitive stimulation in "disadvantaged", but not necessarily malnourished children, to be task specific and temporary. This generalization would suggest that the lack of success of the Cali group in raising the cognitive performance of their malnourished children to the level of well-nourished controls may not have been due to either poor techniques or to any special effect of malnutrition, but rather to the sad conclusion that short bouts of intellectual stimulation in the life of children are not sufficient to produce sustained improvement in intellectual ability.

There are two important ramifications of this conclusion for future research on "the roles of early nutrition and environment in producing healthy, productive citizens". The first point is that the temporary nature of cognitive intervention programmes suggests that we may have overemphasized the permanence of the early environment. If good experience is only temporary, so might be the effects of a bad experience, even an experience with malnutrition. Such a view suggests an optimistic prognosis for children who have suffered from malnutrition.

However, such an optimistic prognosis must be tempered by the other ramification of the "Cali experience" and other studies of cognitive intervention: in order to produce sustained cognitive growth in disadvantaged children, it is necessary to maintain the conditions for optimal growth. Such conditions may be economically and politically unfeasible at the present time in most areas of the world. But this might be the most important lesson learned from the Cali experience.

1. Seligman (1975).

Index